D0292419

Psoriasis

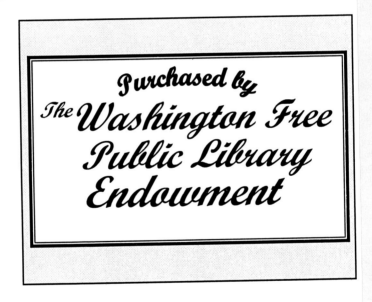

Psoriasis

Dr. Richard G.B. Langley

SECOND EDITION

KEY PORTER BOOKS

Library and Archives Canada Cataloguing in Publication

Langley, Richard G. B
     Psoriasis / Richard Langley. — 2nd ed.

ISBN 978-1-55470-250-3.

    1. Psoriasis—Popular works. I. Title.

RL321.L35 2010   616.5'26   C2009-905866-9

THE CANADA COUNCIL | LE CONSEIL DES ARTS
FOR THE ARTS | DU CANADA
SINCE 1957 | DEPUIS 1957

ONTARIO ARTS COUNCIL
CONSEIL DES ARTS DE L'ONTARIO

The publisher gratefully acknowledges the support of the Canada Council for the Arts and the Ontario Arts Council for its publishing program. We acknowledge the support of the Government of Ontario through the Ontario Media Development Corporation's Ontario Book Initiative.

We acknowledge the financial support of the Government of Canada through the Book Publishing Industry Development Program (BPIDP) for our publishing activities.

This book provides general information on health care and is intended to complement, not substitute for, the advice of your doctor. Before starting any medical treatment or medical program, you should consult with your doctor, who can discuss your individual needs and counsel you about symptoms and treatments. This book is not a substitute for medical diagnosis, and you are advised always to consult your doctor for specific information on personal health matters.

Key Porter Books Limited
Six Adelaide Street East, Tenth Floor
Toronto, Ontario
Canada M5C 1H6
www.keyporter.com

Diagrams: Theresa Sackno
Editor: Paula Chabanais

Printed and bound in Canada

10 11 12 13 14 6 5 4 3 2 1

Contents

Acknowledgements

This book would not have been possible without Christine Langley. She has supported and allowed me the time to pursue my passion for the research, teaching, and practice of dermatology. Dr. Ross Langley and Jean Langley have also provided valuable help, and are my mentors and friends. Finally, I am grateful for the professional help of Linda Pruessen and Paula Chabanais at Key Porter Books, and Yolanda Janiga and Amanda Webb, who helped edit the manuscript.

Introduction

Psoriasis, originating from the Greek word psora (meaning "to itch"), is a chronic, incurable, noncontagious skin disease. For centuries, psoriasis was confused with leprosy. Because of the failure to differentiate between these diseases, people with psoriasis could experience humiliation and abandonment by their family and community.

In the nineteenth century, Dr. Hebra and Dr. Kaposi realized that leprosy was different from psoriasis and helped classify the latter as a distinct medical disease. Since then, scientists have been trying to find the root cause of the disease, effective and safe treatments, and, most importantly, a cure.

Affecting approximately 1–3 percent of the population, psoriasis is one of the most common skin disorders. It can appear at any age and is one of the most common reasons for office visits to dermatologists.

A dermatologist is a doctor who has undergone extensive specialized training in the diagnosis and treatment of skin diseases after completing medical school. Dermatologists are experts in diagnosing and treating diseases of the skin, hair, and nails such as psoriasis. Many psoriasis patients are either dissatisfied or frustrated with their treatments given that psoriasis is currently an incurable disease that can recur after treatment. It is hoped that this book will provide some help and guidance to these patients, and outline some of the promising new treatments for psoriasis.

In the past decade, scientists have gained a better understanding of the disease process of psoriasis. As such, new specific, rational therapies have been and are being developed, and there is reason for great hope that these therapies will effectively treat patients. We and others have participated in international clinical research trials that have studied new, safe, highly targeted, and effective therapies that are providing new choices for patients in the management of this disease. These therapeutic agents are now finding their way into the clinic and to patients with psoriasis and psoriatic arthritis.

This guide will help educate you, your family, and others about psoriasis. In addition, you will gain greater insight into and understanding of the nature of the disease, its potential treatments, and their benefits and risks. Ultimately, this information will enable those affected to effectively deal with their disease and thereby attain a better quality of life.

ONE

Skin: Our Largest Organ

Normal Skin

Human skin is a complicated, important, and fascinating organ. The skin is the largest organ of your body, covering 10.5–21 square feet (1–2 square meters). It forms a vital boundary separating the outside world from the inside of your body.

The skin is an extremely versatile organ: It is flexible yet waterproof; helps keep you warm and cool; and protects you from the environment, foreign substances, and invading organisms that can cause infections. The skin efficiently helps regulate the body's temperature (like a thermostat in a house). Since the temperature of the external environment is constantly changing, the skin must work constantly, in coordination with specialized areas of the brain, to keep the body's temperature within a narrow set range. The skin is tough enough to protect you from the harsh environment, helps coordinate a complex immune regulation of the skin and body, and provides one of our most delicate functions—the sensation of touch.

The skin is also a selective barrier, preventing toxic substances from entering, while permitting the absorption of certain lubricating oils and medications that can help prevent certain diseases (heart attacks and motion sickness), help people avoid smoking and pregnancy, and facilitate hormone replacement. The skin is clearly a dynamic, versatile, and important organ.

Our Skin as a House

It is easier to understand the normal appearance and function of the skin if we compare it to a house and the earth on which that house rests. For example, at its most basic level a house can be considered to comprise two parts: the house itself and the earth it rests on. A two-storey house has a basement and two floors (see illustration). The basement, or foundation, of the house rests on the earth. The house itself consists of bricks and a roof. The bricks are joined together by cement.

Normal Skin Compared to a House

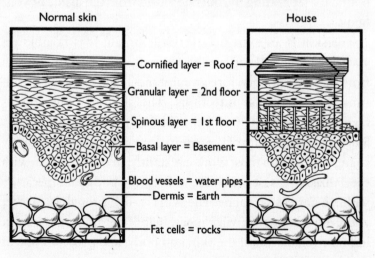

Normal skin   House

- Cornified layer = Roof
- Granular layer = 2nd floor
- Spinous layer = 1st floor
- Basal layer = Basement
- Blood vessels = water pipes
- Dermis = Earth
- Fat cells = rocks

The skin, like a house, is also divided into two parts: the outer, thinner portion called the *epidermis* (which we can think of as our house) and the inner, thicker layer called the *dermis* (which we can think of as the ground or earth). Just as a house rests on the earth for stability, the epidermis rests on top of the dermis.

If the house consists of bricks, cement, and a roof, the skin also has "bricks," "cement," and a "roof." The outer layer of the skin (epidermis) is composed of so-called "bricks," which we call skin cells or keratinocytes. Just as bricks are joined using cement, skin cells or keratinocytes are joined together by small attachments called desmosomes. As cement keeps the bricks together as a continuous layer, desmosomes join the skin cells as a continuous layer.

Getting to Know the House (Epidermis)

Let's now examine the outer layer of skin a little closer.

Just as a house consists of a basement, two floors, and a roof, the epidermis consists of a basement, two floors, and a roof. The "basement" of the skin is called the basal layer. As the basement of the house rests on the earth, the basal layer of the skin rests on the dermis. The two "floors" of the epidermis, in order, are the spinous and granular layers. The "roof" of the epidermis is called the cornified layer.

If we look closely at the house illustration on page 4, we will see that the bricks that form the house consist of different shapes on the different floors. In our skin, the cells that form the outer layer of the skin also change shape in the different layers. The basal layer comprises column-shaped cells, the first and second floors have more round-shaped cells, and the cornified layer of the skin has flat, shingle-like cells.

Basal Layer (Basement)

The bottom layer of the epidermis is the basal layer, which sits right on the dermis. It is a single layer of cuboidal-shaped cells that continuously divide to make skin cells (keratinocytes).

This is similar to the basement of the house, which rests on the earth.

Spinous Layer (First Floor)
The layer of cells above the basal layer is the spinous layer. The skin cells in this layer are more rounded and are pushed upward to the next layer (granular layer).

Granular Layer (Second Floor)
In the next layer, called the granular layer, skin cells stop dividing, their nuclei (the heart of the cell holding all genetic information) start degenerating, and they die. The granular layer is named for the granules present, which contain a specific substance that helps make the skin waterproof. Lipids (fats) and other proteins are also found in this layer.

Our Skin as a House

Layer of house	Layer of skin
• roof	• cornified layer
• second floor	• granular layer
• first floor	• spinous layer
• basement	• basal layer
• earth	• dermis

Cornified Layer (Roof)
The final and outermost layer of the skin is the cornified layer, which consists of flat, dead cells that resemble the shape of the shingles on a roof. This is the layer of skin we see. The cornified layer derives its name from the Latin word for "horn." This layer is horn-like as it consists of dead cells of the epidermis, averaging about twenty cells deep. This creates a tough, protective barrier. The cornified layer sheds every two weeks.

The epidermis is the thinnest layer of the skin, measuring

about 0.4 inch (1 millimeter), or the thickness of several sheets of paper. The thickness varies on different parts of the body. The epidermis is the thickest on the palms of the hands and soles of the feet, and thinnest on the eyelids.

One difference between the house and normal skin is that, unlike the basement of the house, the basal layer of the skin is not flat. It has projections downward called rete ridges (see illustration). (We could think of this as the foundation of a house that has leaked and created lumps in the floor!)

Dermis (Earth)

The epidermis (house) rests on the dermis (earth). Compared to the epidermis, the dermis is thicker and contains nerves, blood vessels, oil (sebaceous) glands, and sweat glands. The dermis is comprised mostly of a strong protein called collagen and a flexible, elastic protein called elastin. These proteins allow the skin to bend and return to its normal shape.

Below the epidermis and dermis is the subcutaneous layer. The main component of this layer is fat, which insulates and protects muscle, bones, and internal organs. Fat is also a reserve source of energy.

Building Our House

Just as a bricklayer would build a house from the basement up, the skin is also built from the basal layer up. The basal layer is where cells divide, supplying the epidermis with new cells every day. New cells are pushed up through the epidermis, and change from column-shaped cells to rounded cells to flat cells. In the cornified layer, the flat skin cells slough off. The entire cycle of growth takes about twenty-eight days.

TWO

What Is Psoriasis?

Psoriasis is a chronic (long-lasting and recurring) inflammatory, noncontagious skin disease, characterized by itchy, thick, raised, red areas of skin covered with silvery-white scales. Psoriatic lesions are most commonly found on the elbows, knees, scalp, and lower back, although any part of the body can be affected, including the fingernails and toenails. Affecting 1–3 percent of the world's population, psoriasis is one of the most common skin disorders.

Psoriasis can vary in presentation and severity. The majority of patients (approximately 80–90 percent) present with relatively mild disease with only limited involvement of the skin, which can be controlled with topical creams. It is important to recognize that even though psoriasis might involve only limited areas of the body, it can still pose a significant burden on patients' lives. This fact was emphasized recently when a major conclusion of a consensus meeting of the American Academy of Dermatology stated that it is important for doctors to not rely only on the *amount* or *area* of a patient's psoriasis when determining the severity of the disease and treatment, but also to take into account the effect the disease has on the patient's quality of life.

Approximately 15–30 percent of psoriasis patients experience arthritis or joint inflammation, which can range in severity from mild to disabling. When severe, psoriatic arthritis can limit a person's ability to walk or work.

Psoriasis can be intensely itchy and have a burning sensation. The disease can cause patients great discomfort, pain, and emotional distress. Depending on the severity, psoriasis can affect relationships and the ability to work or enjoy leisure activities. For example, parents with tender lesions on their hands might find it difficult to care for their babies; patients with painful pustules on their hands or feet can find themselves unable to work with their hands or walk; and food handlers are constantly faced with the question: "Is that contagious?" Teens are often embarrassed by their blemished skin and are unwilling to wear shorts in gym class or during the summer. These limitations can affect both their psychosocial development and ability to enjoy normal healthy activities. In short, psoriasis can have a profound negative physical and psychological impact on patients and their families.

Patients who have more limited disease, however, might not experience much discomfort or be emotionally distressed by its appearance. There are even patients who have extensive areas of their bodies affected but who are not physically or emotionally uncomfortable to any great degree.

Signs and Symptoms

Psoriasis most commonly appears as red, raised, dry scaly areas of the skin. In addition, nail changes such as deformity and crumbling of the nail plate can occur. Arthritis can also be present with joint swelling, tenderness, and stiffness.

The physical appearance and symptoms of psoriasis vary depending on the type of psoriasis and the severity of the disease. The appearance can also vary from person to person, and psoriasis lesions can differ in size from less than an inch to over an inch (several millimeters to several centimeters).

A lesion that is less than 3/8 inch (1 centimeter) in diameter (and is raised above the surface of the skin) is called a papule, and a raised lesion that is greater than 3/8 inch (1 centimeter) in diameter is called a plaque. Some people can have pustules present on the palms and soles or on other areas of the body. Psoriasis can be localized on the elbows and knees, or widespread, covering the entire body.

Types of Psoriasis
There are five different types of psoriasis:
- plaque-type psoriasis
- guttate psoriasis
- inverse psoriasis
- erythrodermic psoriasis
- pustular psoriasis

Each type has its own unique characteristics; some types can occur alone or coincide with other forms. Therapy can differ for each; some therapies are briefly outlined in Chapters 8–12, which focus on the safety and benefits of various treatments.

Plaque-Type Psoriasis
The most common form of psoriasis is known as plaque-type psoriasis (or *psoriasis vulgaris*). As previously explained, the term "plaque" is used to describe a raised area of skin that is greater than 3/8 inch (1 centimeter) in diameter. By definition, many of the areas affected are greater than that in diameter, although smaller areas of raised skin less than 3/8 inch (1 centimeter) (papules) might be present. Smaller papules may join

to form a larger plaque. The affected area is usually raised, red, and scaly. The lesions are usually well defined, meaning that the border between involved skin and uninvolved skin is remarkably sharp. The lesions of psoriasis are normally round to oval in shape. Scales can appear as silvery-white and powdery, and in some cases can be quite thick, even resembling an oyster shell (ostraceous). Scales can flake or peel off in thin transparent sheets. Plaque-type psoriasis occurs in 80–90 percent of all cases and tends to persist for long periods. It affects mostly the elbows, knees, scalp, and lower back (see illustration on page 12). It can, however, involve any part of the body.

The condition commonly appears in a symmetrical pattern (e.g., if the right elbow is affected, the left elbow might also be affected) and can also involve the scalp. When the scalp is affected, it can be intensely itchy. Scalp psoriasis can be one of the most frustrating and difficult areas to treat.

Plaque-type psoriasis can affect the genitals. Men are more likely to be affected in this location than women. Genital lesions can cause embarrassment during sexual relations, especially if the penis is affected. Affected areas of skin can become redder and more noticeable after intercourse. It is important that affected people are aware that lesions are not contagious, so they can reassure themselves and advise sexual partners.

Often patients are too embarrassed to tell their doctors that genital areas are affected. However, it is important to tell your doctor as there are treatments to help control psoriasis in these locations. Topical corticosteroids are usually effective in treating genital psoriasis. However, thinning of the skin (atrophy) and stretch marks (striae) can occur when potent steroids are applied for prolonged periods to such sensitive areas. In general, lower potency topical steroids are used in areas where the skin is thin. Higher potency topical steroids generally should be avoided on the genitals.

Newer, nonsteroidal treatments known as calcineurin inhibitors or topical immunomodulators (tacrolimus/protopic 0.1 percent and 0.3 percent and pimecrolimus/elidel 1 percent cream) have been used in psoriasis. Calcineurin inhibitors offer the advantage of being steroid-free, with no risk of stretch marks or thinning of the skin. Applying anthralin or coal tar products to genital lesions is not recommended as they can cause irritation.

Common Distribution Patterns of Psoriasis

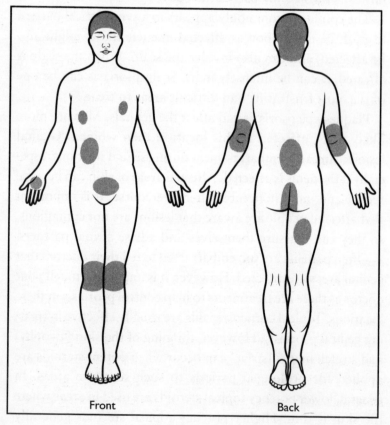

Front   Back

The palms of the hands and soles of the feet can also be affected, although less frequently in plaque-type psoriasis. The lesions can be commonly noted on the pressure-bearing areas of the hands and feet.

Guttate Psoriasis

The Latin word *gutta*, meaning "droplet," describes the physical appearance of the lesions in this type of psoriasis. In guttate psoriasis, patients often describe the sudden appearance of small (1/8 inch/2–3 millimeters in diameter), raised, scaling bumps. Classically, guttate psoriasis can start in childhood or teenage years after streptococcal infections of the throat (streptococcal pharyngitis) or tonsillitis. A sudden flare-up of numerous tiny red, raised bumps (papules) covering large areas of the body can arise two to four weeks after the illness. The number of lesions can increase and spread rapidly over the trunk, arms, legs, and sometimes the face.

In children, an episode of guttate psoriasis usually clears up after the initial episode and does not recur. However, chronic psoriasis can follow. In adults, guttate psoriasis can develop into plaque-type psoriasis. Phototherapy (see Chapter 10) is particularly effective for guttate psoriasis.

Inverse Psoriasis

Inverse psoriasis (also known as flexural psoriasis) affects areas where the body folds, such as the skin in the armpits, groin, under the breasts, and in the perianal location. This type of psoriasis usually occurs in conjunction with plaque-type psoriasis, but can also occur on its own. It differs from other types of psoriasis because rather than appearing scaly, the skin is smooth, moist, and salmon-colored. Inverse psoriasis can be confused with a yeast (candida) or fungal infection (jock itch).

People with inverse psoriasis can feel extremely uncomfortable because their skin is often raw, tender, or itchy, which is most distressing for those affected as scratching these areas in public is embarrassing. Sweating can irritate the skin further. Inverse psoriasis can usually be controlled with topical corticosteroids. A mild to mid-potency topical steroid is usually tried first as the skin in these locations is thinner and more likely to develop local side effects from topical steroids (thinning of the skin, stretch marks). As noted earlier, a new kind of topical nonsteroidal therapy is now available and is also used to treat psoriasis in these locations. The new therapies are available in cream formulations.

Erythrodermic Psoriasis

Erythrodermic psoriasis is a severe form of psoriasis. Also known as exfoliative psoriasis—because scaly lesions cover all or almost all of the body and the skin can be scaling and peeling—it is characterized by widespread, extremely red, itchy, and swollen skin. For some, the skin can be very red with minimal scaling. In areas of raw skin, pustules might be present and pus can ooze from these lesions. The eyes, the lining of the mouth, and the inside of the nose can also be affected.

Erythrodermic psoriasis usually appears in one of two forms. First, a chronic, long-standing plaque-type psoriasis may gradually progress so that increasing areas of skin become involved. Second, erythrodermic psoriasis can occur in people with unstable psoriasis and can be triggered by several factors, including illness, emotional stress, alcoholism, and the withdrawal of potent topical, oral, and/or injected corticosteroids.

Those with erythrodermic psoriasis can be quite sick (possibly with fevers and chills), are prone to infection in the involved skin, and might have difficulty maintaining normal levels of fluids and body temperature. As a result of the increased volume of blood flowing through severely inflamed skin, the patient can develop an increased heart rate, particularly those who are elderly or who have prior heart disease, and this can ultimately lead to heart failure.

Those presenting with erythrodermic psoriasis should be referred to a dermatologist. Basic principles of care include maintaining normal levels of fluids and the liberal use of a moisturizer and/or topical steroids. In order to restore normal levels of fluids and nutrients, some cases will require hospitalization. Once a patient is stabilized, typical treatments such as topical therapy, phototherapy, oral medications, or biologic therapy can be used to control the disease (see Chapters 8–12).

Pustular Psoriasis
Pustular psoriasis is characterized by the appearance of small blister-like areas on the skin. Pustular psoriasis can be separated into two forms: localized (often only the hands and feet) and generalized (extensive areas of the body). Localized, or palmoplantar pustulosis (PPP), is the most common pustular variant. Those with generalized pustular psoriasis (GPP) are among the most seriously ill and will usually require hospitalization until the psoriasis is controlled.

The blister-like lesions of pustular psoriasis are usually small and raised. These lesions are filled with noninfectious pus (white blood cells, cellular debris, and dead tissue) and are surrounded by reddened skin. The skin may be painful, which makes manual labor or walking difficult. Pustular psoriasis can be triggered by infections, stress, or certain medications. Smoking may also play a role.

Psoriasis at Special Sites

Scalp Psoriasis

The scalp is one of the most common and persistent areas affected by psoriasis (occurring in about 50 percent of all patients) and can be one of the most difficult places to treat. The scales on the scalp can be thick and silvery-white, and can stick together tightly to form dense crusts that can be very itchy. Picking at the scales and scratching the scalp can worsen the psoriasis.

Scalp psoriasis can be localized, involving only a few discrete areas or can affect the entire scalp. The lesions often appear behind the ears and along the hairline, but can spread beyond the hairline. If the ear canal is affected and accumulates enough scales, hearing may be impaired. Hair loss is uncommon because psoriasis does not affect the hair root, but in severe cases hair loss can occur. Hair usually regrows once the psoriasis is controlled.

Mild outbreaks of scalp psoriasis that remain hidden by the hair might not be noticed by an observer; however, severe forms can be extremely itchy and highly visible. Silvery-white scales (resembling dandruff) flake onto shoulders and collar, which can be embarrassing and emotionally stressful for the patient. Successful treatment is important to minimize the emotional stresses and physical discomforts.

Grace is a forty-eight-year-old public relations specialist, with a bubbly, enthusiastic, humorous manner that is highly infectious. She is an active woman and married with two children, both of whom are in university. Approximately two years ago she came to see me with a history of having an "awful head." This problem involved significant itching, and constant scaling and shedding from her scalp that was visible on her clothing, particularly with darker colors. This was making her self-conscious, and she was also finding the condition embarrassing as she would tend to scratch her itchy scalp. It was clear that the condition was causing her significant discomfort. She described a problem of thickening toenails, which she attributed to a "fungus." She had treated herself with multiple over-the-counter dandruff shampoos without any effect. There was no family history of psoriasis.

When I examined Grace's scalp, virtually the entire area was covered with a thick, white, adherent scale. It was evident that the scalp was quite inflamed and red. She had a number of areas that were open and bleeding due to scratching in an attempt to alleviate the itching. The nails of both big toes were yellow, thick, and discolored. Otherwise she was completely healthy.

After examining Grace, it was clear to me that she had scalp psoriasis. I suspected that her "fungal" nails were in fact also a manifestation of psoriasis. I took fungal cultures of her nails, which were negative, a result that supported a diagnosis of psoriasis.

I explained to Grace that while scalp psoriasis can be both challenging to treat and a recurrent problem, we should be able to get it under much better control, providing a reduction in her symptoms and her social concerns. I discussed with her the need to reduce the amount of scaling on her scalp and the inflammation or redness that was causing her such intense itching. For this, I used a topical lotion for the scalp, which combined salicylic acid with a topical steroid. By using this combination, we removed the scale, as well as reduced the inflammation and the itch. I also recommended that she use a tar-based shampoo on a regular basis. This can also help reduce the scaling and control her symptoms.

When I saw her a month later, she was delighted. For the first time, she had significant control of her symptoms, her "awful head" was now controlled with minimal scaling on her clothing, and there was no significant itch. At this point, I recommended discontinuing the topical salicylic acid–steroid lotion and using only a mild topical steroid as she still had some mild inflammation or redness in the scalp. Given that the scaling had been reduced, there was no need for the salicylic acid, which was initially helpful in enhancing the penetration of the topical steroid and reducing the scaling. If used after the scaling is gone, it can be irritating to the scalp. I now see her only occasionally as she is able to control her symptoms with a tar-based shampoo and with as-needed use of the topical steroid.

Treatment of scalp psoriasis is challenging, but there are many therapies that can help. Sometimes, the best treatments are arrived at by trial and error, so it is important to be patient when treating and awaiting results. The following are some common forms of treatment.

Anthralin: Anthralin can reduce the turnover of skin cells that cause the excessive buildup of scale, and reduce inflammation. As a result, it can be highly effective in treating scalp psoriasis. However, anthralin can be messy and cause staining of the skin, blond or gray hair, and clothing.

Anthralin can be applied directly to the skin for short periods (short contact anthralin therapy or SCAT) of 15–30 minutes. It should then be washed off to prevent irritation. Lower strengths of anthralin can be used and left on the skin for longer periods.

If your skin is tender and sore from psoriasis, anthralin might not be the best choice as it can cause irritation of the scalp.

Salicylic acid: Salicylic acid (keratolytic) is an ingredient in certain over-the-counter shampoos. It is helpful in removing excessive scales, which in turn allows for the penetration of other medications (such as steroids) into the site of inflammation. Salicylic acid can be mixed in low concentrations in mineral oil or provided in combination with a topical steroid (betamethasone dipropionate/salicylic acid) or combined with tar in a shampoo.

Shampoos: Shampoos that contain active ingredients such as tar, salicylic acid, zinc pyrithione, or selenium sulfide can be very helpful in reducing the scaling and thickness of scalp psoriasis. Recently, shampoos that contain steroids have been developed and can be quite helpful for patients.

Topical steroids: Steroid-containing scalp preparations can be very effective in reducing redness (inflammation) in psoriasis of the scalp. Steroids are usually prescribed either as a lotion, solution, or foam for hair-bearing areas (creams and ointments are difficult to apply to the hair-bearing scalp, often causing the hair to become matted). Alcohol-based lotions can cause stinging, so a water-based lotion can be substituted (amcinonide).

Topical vitamin D analogues (calcipotriol): Topical calcipotriol (Dovonex®, Daivonex®) scalp solution can be used alone or in combination with other topical treatments. Recently, a combination of topical steroids (betamethasone dipropionate) and calcipotriol (Xamiol®) was approved for use in the treatment of scalp psoriasis. The combination of these agents was shown to be very effective, leading to excellent results in 56–83 percent of patients.

Nail Psoriasis

Psoriasis can affect the nails in up to 50 percent of patients, and this number can be higher if psoriatic arthritis is present. Some people might have only nail psoriasis with no apparent skin changes on the rest of the body. Psoriasis of the fingernails is more common than psoriasis of the toenails. Several changes can occur in the nail with psoriasis.

Discoloration: The nail can develop a yellow-brown discoloration that might involve the entire nail. The discoloration can also occur in only one or a few localized areas in a spot-like manner and resemble an oil droplet.

Nail Changes in Psoriasis

- Deformation: Change in nail shape
- Discoloration: Change in color of the nail to yellow-brown
- Hyperkeratosis: Thickening of the nail plate
- Onycholysis: Lifting up of the nail
- Pitting: Shallow depressions in nail plate—"dents"

Fungal infections of the nails: A fungal infection of the nails (which may occur along with nail psoriasis) can also cause thickening of the nails. It is not uncommon for nail psoriasis to be misdiagnosed as a fungal infection. Fungal infections should be treated, if possible, because they can worsen psoriasis.

In order to make a proper diagnosis, a doctor takes nail clippings and a fungal culture. Once an infection is confirmed, treatment is most effective with oral antifungals. Topical treatment of nail fungus is usually ineffective, although new nail lacquers may be effective in certain patients.

Hyperkeratosis or onycholysis: The affected nail might thicken or lift away from the skin attached to the nail. When the nail lifts away from the nail bed it is called onycholysis (see illustration). It usually begins at the edge or at the end of the nail and may continue backward under the nail until it is completely loosened from the nail bed.

Pitting (see illustration below): The most common finding in nail psoriasis is pitting. Pits are shallow depressions or dents, less than 1/32 inch (1 millimeter) in diameter, and look like pinholes. They can affect all nails, some, or none.

Other changes: Other changes in nail psoriasis include depressions in the nail, or roughness and grooving of the nail. If severe, patients may lose their nails, making it difficult to grasp

Nail Changes in Psoriasis

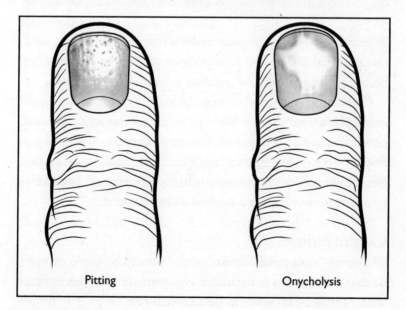

Pitting   Onycholysis

Pitting (left): refers to shallow depressions that look like pin holes in the nail.
Onycholysis (right): refers to lifting of the nail plate.

objects. Bacterial and fungal infections may also develop in a nail already affected with psoriasis.

Nail psoriasis is difficult to treat; both patients and dermatologists are often disappointed with the results. Treatment can take prolonged periods before improvement is seen. Topical treatments are generally ineffective in treating nail disease.

Systemic treatments (oral or injectable medications—see Chapter 11) can improve nail psoriasis. Methotrexate (Rheumatrex®) and cyclosporine (Sandimmune®) can be particularly effective, but it is important to compare the risks of therapy with the benefits of treatment. Recently, infliximab (Remicade®) has been demonstrated to be very effective in treating nail psoriasis. If only the nails are affected, systemic medications are rarely used because the risks of therapy usually outweigh the benefits. If extensive areas of the body are affected, systemic therapy may be a reasonable option. Also, intralesional injections of corticosteroids can be effective, but because it is painful, few patients tolerate this treatment.

If you receive an oral or injectable medication and the psoriasis elsewhere on the body shows improvement, the nail psoriasis may also improve. Scarring or permanent nail loss does not occur in nail psoriasis even in the most severe cases, but it can take six to twelve months for a fingernail, and twelve to eighteen months for a toenail to be replaced.

Comorbidities

The term "comorbid" describes the presence of one or more diseases in addition to the underlying primary disorder. Patients with psoriasis can be at increased risk for developing a number of other important medical conditions. These diseases or comorbid conditions are often chronic (long-lasting), and can have a significant impact on patients' quality of life, productivity at work, and general health. Comorbidities in patients with psoriasis can include arthritis (psoriatic arthritis), depression, inflammatory bowel disease, lymphoma, and the so-called metabolic syndrome (the coexistence of heart disease, high blood pressure, and obesity).

Heart Disease

Several research studies have reported the association of ischemic (ischemia describes decreased blood supply to an organ, tissue, or part caused by constriction or obstruction of the blood vessels) heart disease or coronary artery disease and psoriasis. Several large studies, which compared a group of patients with psoriasis and a group of patients without psoriasis, found that in the group with psoriasis there were increased rates of obesity, high blood pressure (hypertension), and heart disease. In medicine, the term often used to describe the grouping of high blood pressure, heart disease, and obesity is "the metabolic syndrome." These are recognized risk factors for heart disease.

Depression or Depression Symptoms

Psoriasis can have a significant negative impact on patients' quality of life and lead to depressive symptoms (see Chapter 7). In several large clinical studies of patients who undergo treatment with a biologic therapy, almost a third were found to have symptoms of depression at baseline. Not surprisingly, other findings showed that the degree of depression is related to the severity of psoriasis, and that patients with severe disease were more likely to have thoughts of suicide.

Psoriatic Arthritis

Psoriatic arthritis is one of the most common associations with psoriasis, occurring in approximately a third of patients with psoriasis (see Chapter 5).

Cancer

Several studies have shown that psoriasis and treatments for psoriasis are associated with an increased risk of cancer. For example, skin cancer, particularly squamous cell cancer, has been associated with psoriasis patients, particularly those who have received phototherapy. Lymphoma (malignant tumors) has also been recognized as a health concern that is associated with psoriasis. *An increase in the risk of lymphomas in psoriasis patients, particularly those with more severe psoriasis, has been documented. It is not clear yet what part, if any, of this risk is due to medications used to treat psoriasis compared to the risk, if any, of having the skin disease psoriasis.*

What Can You Do about the Possibility of Comorbidities?

Be encouraged by the fact that many of the risk factors, particularly the cardiac risk factors, can be modified. Weight loss, exercise, reduction of stress, and cessation of smoking are key components to help reduce the risk of cardiac disease. Talk to your physician to discuss particular measures. Recent and ongoing research suggests that some of the associated health concerns, such as depression and risk of cancer, may be reduced by the effective treatment of psoriasis. All these findings go a long way to emphasize the importance of treating a chronic inflammatory disease, such as psoriasis, as these diseases may have an effect on your general health. In this sense, psoriasis is truly more than just "skin deep."

THREE

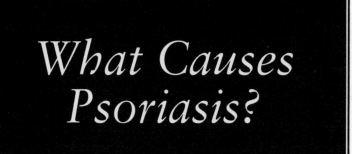

What Causes Psoriasis?

In the past decade, there have been many advances in our understanding of how psoriasis might develop and how it can be treated. The question remains: Why does it occur? Psoriasis is a complex disease that is caused by several factors. Although there is no known single cause for psoriasis, it is clear that genetics, the skin cells (keratinocytes), environmental factors, and the immune system play central roles in causing this disease. Psoriasis has a strong genetic component, and there are multiple genes that likely need environmental triggers to activate psoriasis. There are many theories as to why psoriasis occurs in susceptible people, but no one has been able to pinpoint the exact cause. We now understand, however, that there are several key steps in the process, and that the immune system plays a critical role.

Traditionally, a leading theory proposed that psoriasis was caused by an abnormality in the outer layer of the skin (epidermis), and that the unrestricted growth of the epidermis led to an increased growth rate of these cells—in psoriasis the skin cells grow more rapidly, often during three to five days (as opposed to the normal twenty-eight-day cycle); they divide much faster than normal skin cells, and the number of cells multiplying is doubled, which, in turn, leads to thickening and scaling skin. In other words, it was believed that somehow the skin of people with psoriasis was different and, therefore, led to the disease.

While these understandings are important, increasing attention has focused on the immune system as pivotal in the development of psoriasis. Specifically, the red, thick, and scaly changes seen in the skin occur *in reaction to* a faulty signal from the immune system to the skin. In other words, the inflamed plaques of psoriasis arise from a series of abnormal reactions in the skin.

Normal Skin versus Psoriatic Skin

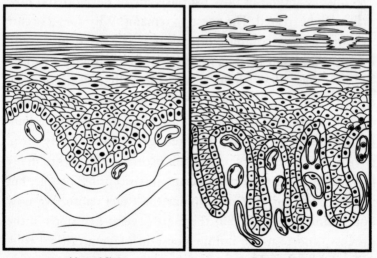

Normal Skin   Psoriatic skin

The Immune System

The immune system is the first line of defense that guards our body from foreign substances. In the last two decades, compelling scientific information has suggested that the immune system is the most important factor in causing psoriasis. One important observation that was helpful in developing this concept came about when a chance clinical observation revealed an improvement in psoriasis symptoms in patients being treated with cyclosporine for their arthritis. Although cyclosporine was not being used for the patient's psoriasis, the unexpected improvement helped open the door to using cyclosporine for psoriasis and, in part, to new understandings about the causes of psoriasis.

Cyclosporine is a drug used to prevent the rejection of transplanted organs. It acts by suppressing the immune system (see Chapter 11), an effect that led to improvements in psoriasis. Thus, a link between the immune system and psoriasis was made. This discovery was one of the first indications that psoriasis was caused, in part, by imbalances in the immune system. Since that observation was made, scientists have been accumulating evidence that established that the immune system plays a central role in the development of psoriasis, partially by sending a faulty signal to the outer layer of the skin (epidermis), which causes it to thicken.

The significance of these discoveries cannot be overstated. They led to a clearer understanding of the exact way psoriasis occurs, thereby providing scientists with the opportunity to develop new medications that can specifically target the immune system and ultimately allow us to use new medicines to effectively treat this capricious disease.

The Immune System and Disease

When our immune system functions normally it is able to effectively protect us against invading microorganisms, such as bacteria, viruses, and fungi, and foreign substances called antigens, as well as to prevent the occurrence of cancer and other diseases. The importance of an intact, functioning immune system can be readily appreciated when we visualize what happens if this system is disturbed. For example, individuals with *inherited* abnormalities of the immune system are prone to frequent infections and cancers (see sidebar on page 29).

In addition, the immune system is able to survey the skin and other organs, detect precancerous and cancerous changes, and possibly prevent the development of certain cancers. People with *acquired* immune deficiencies, such as acquired immune deficiency syndrome (AIDS), are prone to serious infections and cancers.

While a decrease in our immune system can make us susceptible to diseases, an increase or overstimulation of our immune system can lead to a type of disease called autoimmune disease. An autoimmune disease is caused, in part, by an overstimulation of our body's immune defenses, in which our immune cells start attacking our healthy cells. This happens in part because our immune cells fail to recognize our healthy cells, mistaking them for a foreign substance and attacking them.

Immunology for Everyone

A key component in the immune system is a group of cells called *white blood cells*, which help defend the body against foreign invaders and microorganisms. One type of white blood cell that is believed to be of crucial importance in causing psoriasis is the T-lymphocyte.

The T-lymphocytes are very smart cells because they have terrific memories. In fact, once they are exposed to a foreign substance, they remember it forever. With subsequent exposures, the T-lymphocytes will recognize the substance and multiply to attack it. Hence, they are known as memory T-cells.

While T-cells have great memories for foreign substances, they need a teacher. That teacher is known as an antigen presenting cell (APC), which does exactly what its name says: It presents antigen (foreign substances) to the T-cell and teaches

The Boy in the Bubble

In the 1970s, the unfortunate true story of David Vetter was widely known. David was born with a rare inherited disorder known as severe combined immunodeficiency (SCID). SCID involves severe defects in the immune system. As a result, David was susceptible to any germs around him, as he basically had no immune system to fight them. David lived for nearly thirteen years inside a sealed plastic bubble, which protected him from infections. His room was sealed and his food specially prepared. His only human contact came in the form of gloved hands.

This story inspired songs (Paul Simon's "The Boy in a Bubble") and movies (*Bubble Boy*). Fortunately, there are now treatments for this potentially devastating condition. David's story illustrates the important role of the immune system in defending us against foreign microorganisms such as bacteria, viruses, and fungi.

the T-cell about the antigen. The T-cell, with its fantastic memory, will then remember that foreign substance in future encounters. T-cells naturally circulate throughout the body looking for antigens. The presence of the antigen, usually an outside invader, such as a virus or bacteria, activates the T-cell, which then initiates an immune response to neutralize the antigen.

In psoriasis, activated T-cells accumulate in the outer layer (epidermis) and inner layer (dermis) of the skin, where they reproduce at a rapid rate due to chemicals called cytokines, such as tumor necrosis factor-alpha (TNF-alpha), which sends a faulty message to the skin, causing the skin cells to grow and divide more rapidly and resulting in the thick, scaly skin of psoriasis. The reason this happens and the exact process continue to be the focus of intense scientific interest and research. It is becoming increasingly clear that certain interleukins, interleukin-23 (IL-23) and interleukin-22 (IL-22), and new types of recently described T-cell (T-helper 17) are of central importance in the development of psoriasis.

Interleukin-12, interleukin-22, and interleukin-23 are recognized as important chemical messengers in the cause of psoriasis. These chemicals, or cytokines, have been shown to induce the changes in the skin that are consistent with psoriasis, both in animals and human experiments.

Researchers in the mid-1990s proved that T-cells in the skin release specific cytokines (proteins) that are capable of causing skin cells to grow. Researchers are still carefully examining the process to determine the specific antigen that activates the immune system and fuels the entire process—the so-called key to psoriasis.

Taken together, this summarizes our current understanding of the immune mechanisms causing psoriasis. This has taken scientists more than twenty years to understand. These understandings have provided important insight into permitting the development of new medicines to treat these immune defects and improve psoriasis (see Chapter 12).

Who Is Most at Risk?

Psoriasis is most commonly diagnosed between the ages of 15 and 35, but it can occur at birth or, less often, in the elderly. The average age of onset in males is 29, and in females, 27. A second peak can occur in the mid-50s. About 10–15 percent of all cases occur in children under the age of 10. Men and women are affected equally. Although anyone can develop psoriasis, the incidences are much lower in West Africans, African Americans, Japanese, Inuit, and Native Americans, a fact that led researchers to believe the cause of psoriasis might involve genetic and environmental factors or triggers.

Genetics

A family history of psoriasis has long been known as a risk factor for developing this disease. Approximately one-third of patients have a family history of psoriasis. If a first-degree relative has psoriasis, such as a sibling or parent, then there is a 10–20 percent chance of the child developing psoriasis as well. If both parents have psoriasis, the risk of their child developing psoriasis is 50 percent. These statistics strongly suggest that genes or genetics play an important and central role in causing psoriasis.

A gene is a part of the DNA (deoxyribonucleic acid) that contains information you inherit. This information includes the color of your hair and eyes, and whether you are susceptible to certain diseases. Researchers are still uncertain which specific genes are involved or exactly how the environment plays a role in triggering psoriasis. In fact, it may be that several genes are required to cause psoriasis.

One of the strongest indications that psoriasis has a genetic basis comes from studies of identical twins. Identical twins have all the same genes. Fraternal twins, however, share only some of the same genes. In identical twins, chances are three times greater that psoriasis will be present in both siblings, compared to fraternal twins. Even if multiple genes are required to cause psoriasis, this finding is important in indicating a genetic basis.

Triggers
While psoriasis has a definite genetic component, environmental factors also play a key role in the onset and severity of disease. Patients with psoriasis might note that they experience a worsening or flare-up of their disease in response to external or internal factors. There are many such factors that can indirectly trigger the onset of psoriasis or aggravate it in someone who is already affected. These include:
• climate
• infection
• medications
• skin injury (Koebner phenomenon)
• stress

Climate
Many patients will experience changes in their condition in different seasons, and typically report that cold weather can worsen their psoriasis, while sunlight is usually beneficial.

Infection
Certain infections, such as streptococcal throat infections, are believed to trigger a flare of psoriasis (See Chapter 2: guttate psoriasis).

Medications
Certain medications have been related to aggravating psoriasis, including antimalarials, beta-blockers, lithium, and interferons. Sudden discontinuation of treatment with cyclosporine, systemic corticosteroids, is known to cause psoriasis flare-ups in some patients. Medications that may induce or worsen psoriasis include:

Antimalarials (used to treat malaria initially and now other conditions such as lupus)
- chloroquine
- hydroxychloroquine
- quinacrine

Beta-blockers (used to treat high blood pressure)
- acebutolol
- atenolol
- metoprolol
- propranolol
- sotalol HCL

Interferons (used to treat hepatitis C, multiple sclerosis, cancer)
- interferon <alpha>
- interferon <gamma>

Lithium carbonate (used to treat manic-depressive disorder)

Skin Injury (Koebner phenomenon)
Psoriasis can occur after injury to the skin. This is known as the Koebner phenomenon. Any picking, scratching, or injuries from cuts, burns, or bruises can trigger the development of new psoriatic lesions at the exact site of injury. This could partly explain why psoriasis can be present over the elbows and knees, where friction and trauma are frequent, or after surgery at the site of a surgical scar.

Stress
Excessive stress can play a role in making psoriasis worse. Stress is a constant feature of modern life, but major events that cause significant stress can cause a flare-up in a patient's psoriasis. For example, sickness, job pressures, the death of a loved one, or relationship breakups are all events that may cause a flare-up in psoriasis.

Stress is not the root cause of psoriasis, but it can aggravate an existing condition or lead to the development of psoriasis in predisposed people. Stress can also delay the healing process. In a study at the University of Manchester (U.K.), it was found that psoriasis patients who worry excessively might experience slower responses to phototherapy than those who do not worry a great deal. The findings revealed that those patients classified as "high-level" worriers took about twice as long to improve than those who were "low-level" worriers.

Other
Other factors that may contribute to psoriasis onset or worsening include smoking (with pustular psoriasis) and alcohol.

FOUR

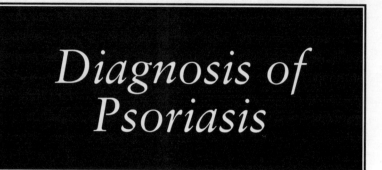

Diagnosis of Psoriasis

With any disease, an accurate diagnosis is the first step in ensuring proper treatment. A doctor makes the diagnosis of psoriasis after she or he has asked a series of questions and carefully examined your skin. In most cases, the physical examination of your skin alone is enough to make the diagnosis. There are a few things doctors will ask when making a diagnosis:

- Is there a family history of psoriasis?
- How long have you had this condition?
- What treatments have you received?
- How effective were they?
- Do you have tender and/or swollen joints (arthritis)?
- Are your fingernails/toenails affected?
- Do you have a history of skin lesions improving in summer and worsening in winter?
- Do you have one or more raised, red, silvery, scaling areas?
- Is the disease in the classic locations with symmetrical involvement of the elbows, knees, lower back, scalp, finger and/or toenails (rough, discolored appearance, often with individual pits in the nail plate)?

As discussed in Chapter 2 there are multiple types of psoriasis, and your doctor will examine you to see which type you have. Also, your doctor might want to see if other body areas are involved, such as the joints (see Chapter 5: "Psoriatic Arthritis").

How Is Psoriasis Diagnosed?

Your doctor will analyze your skin, nails, and scalp in search of signs of psoriasis. The nails show changes in about 50 percent of all cases. There could be pitting, which looks like pinholes in the nail, and/or the nails may be yellowish or thickened, with ridges and scales heaped up at the free edge (see page 21).

If there is still doubt whether psoriasis is present or not, the doctor could:

• perform a biopsy of the skin
• request X-rays, especially when joint pain is apparent
• take blood tests

Let's take a look at these options in more detail.

Biopsy

A skin biopsy is used only in those instances when it is difficult to diagnose the disease. This relatively painless procedure involves numbing a small area of skin with a local anesthetic. A special instrument, called a "punch biopsy," is then rotated on the skin and light pressure applied, removing about a 1/8 inch (3–4 millimeter) piece of skin for testing. Following this procedure, one or two sutures might be used to stitch the skin, and a bandage applied.

The skin sample is then examined under a microscope. A pathologist—a doctor specially trained to examine skin tissue under a microscope—will assist in examining the sample.

Certain characteristics of the analyzed skin will help pathologists determine if psoriasis is the underlying cause.

X-rays

Where there is joint swelling or signs of joint deformity, X-rays can reveal characteristic damage to the joints. If there are signs of arthritis, the family doctor or dermatologist could request a rheumatologist—a specialist in arthritis—to examine the joints and assess the condition further.

Blood Tests

Blood tests may be performed if you have arthritis. A blood test called rheumatoid factor is commonly done to exclude rheumatoid arthritis. Rheumatoid factor is a protein found in the blood of most patients with rheumatoid arthritis. Most patients with psoriatic arthritis test negative for rheumatoid factor. Recently, it has become increasingly clear that psoriasis patients have an increased rate for a number of associated medical conditions, such as high blood pressure, diabetes, and obesity. As a result, your doctor may take your blood pressure, check your blood glucose, and perform a C-reactive protein test, which measures inflammation.

Distinguishing Psoriasis from Other Conditions

The diagnosis of psoriasis is usually straightforward. Still, several conditions can often be confused with psoriasis, eczema, and fungal (tinea) infections being the most common.

Eczema

Eczema differs from psoriasis in several ways.
- When eczema first appears, it is often wet and oozing. Psoriasis is usually dry with thick scales.

- Eczema is often very itchy, whereas psoriasis is often mildly itchy or not itchy at all. Some patients with psoriasis, however, can have itchy lesions.
- Cracks in the skin are often present in eczema.
- Patients with a hereditary form of eczema, called atopic eczema/dermatitis, often have a history of hay fever or asthma.
- Most cases of atopic eczema begin before two years of age, whereas most cases of psoriasis occur in adults.
- Eczema usually lacks the silvery scales of psoriasis.
- When eczema first appears, it is usually difficult to see a clear, well-defined border separating normal skin from eczema. In plaque psoriasis, there is a well-defined border that can usually be clearly distinguished from normal skin.
- Eczema may be confused with psoriasis, particularly if it has been present for several years.
- Hand or foot eczema may resemble psoriasis as the skin can be very thick.
- Eczema patients usually lack the nail changes seen in psoriasis patients.

Characteristic	Eczema	Psoriasis
Common site of involvement	Creases in forearms and behind knees	Elbows, knees and scalp
Itchy	Moderate to severe	Mild to moderate; may be absent
History of asthma	Frequent	Less common

Fungal Infections (Tinea)
- Fungal skin infections (commonly known as ringworm) are infections of the skin and nails that can resemble psoriasis.
- They may cause raised, red, scaly areas of the scalp (tinea capitis), body (tinea corporis), and hands or feet (tinea pedis).
- Fungal skin infections may also involve the nails.

These are several differences between psoriasis and fungal skin infections.

Characteristics	Psoriasis	Fungal Skin Infections
Symmetrical	Yes	No
Silvery scale	Yes	No
Scale absent in center of affected skin	Not often	Often
Culture of the skin	Negative (for fungus)	Positive (for fungus)

To establish a diagnosis, your doctor may take a scraping of the skin or clippings from the nail. These can be examined under a microscope, or cultured, and a diagnosis of fungus can be made, if positive.

Candidiasis

- In the groin or under the breasts, candida infections (caused by yeast) may appear similar to inverse psoriasis.
- Taking a small scraping and examining the skin under the microscope can help distinguish psoriasis from candida infections.

FIVE

Psoriatic Arthritis

Psoriatic arthritis is a chronic (long-term), progressive, inflammatory arthritis (swelling and tenderness of the joints). People with psoriatic arthritis can have swollen, tender joints, as well as nail changes, and the scaly, raised, red skin changes of psoriasis.

Inflammation most commonly involves the joints of the hands, wrists, neck, back, knees, ankles, and feet. The pain and stiffness are usually worse in the morning, or after rest, and can improve with physical activity. The severity can vary from mild disease affecting only a few joints without any noticeable pain to severe disabling and painful arthritis with deformity and destruction of joints. In people with mild arthritis, the condition can remain undiagnosed and might have minimal impact on their quality of life. More severe forms of psoriatic arthritis can occur in people with multiple affected joints (more than four), and in younger, often female patients. Early diagnosis and treatment is important to prevent destruction and deformity of the joints.

In most people, the skin lesions of psoriasis usually occur before arthritis develops. Less commonly, arthritis can occur at the same time or before skin changes occur. In the past, it was believed that approximately 5 percent of patients with psoriasis had psoriatic arthritis. Recent research has determined that approximately 15–30 percent of patients with psoriasis develop psoriatic arthritis.

Psoriatic arthritis belongs to a group of conditions known as seronegative spondyloarthropathies. The term "seronegative" means that the blood (sero) is negative for a certain factor present in rheumatoid arthritis. The blood test is for the rheumatoid factor, which is a protein found in the blood of most patients with another type of arthritis called rheumatoid arthritis. The term "spondylo" means spine, and "arthropathy" means painful, swollen joints. Spondyloarthropathy refers to a group of conditions that share several features, including:

- a pattern of arthritis that affects the spine and extremities
- inflammation of ligaments and tendons
- inflammation of other organs such as the eye
- evidence of a family history of psoriatic arthritis

In the past, psoriatic arthritis may have been underrecognized. Also, accurate data has been difficult to gather because patients with psoriatic arthritis might not feel much pain, so the disease can go unnoticed until it has progressed and there are deformities.

Understanding Arthritis

Arthritis: Inflammation (redness, swelling, and tenderness) of a joint
Monoarthritis: A single joint is affected
Oligoarthritis: Only a few joints are affected
Polyarthritis: Many joints are affected

- Psoriatic arthritis can be a difficult type of arthritis to diagnose, and doctors may misdiagnose psoriatic arthritis for another form of arthritis. There has been a lack of widely accepted criteria for diagnosing psoriatic arthritis.
- New criteria are currently being developed by rheumatologists to assist in diagnosing and assessing psoriatic arthritis.

What Causes Psoriatic Arthritis?

The exact cause of psoriatic arthritis is unknown. Yet, like psoriasis, genetic, environmental, and immunological factors are considered important in the development of psoriatic arthritis.

Genetic Factors

Psoriatic arthritis is more common in those with a family history (particularly in an affected parent or sibling) of the disease.

Environmental Factors

Although the initial event that causes psoriatic arthritis is unknown, trauma and infection are possible triggers for the development of psoriatic arthritis.

Immunological Factors

The immune system is of central importance in the cause of psoriatic arthritis. The activation of the T-cells in the immune system can cause the release of inflammatory messengers called cytokines, which are found in high levels in the joints of patients with psoriatic arthritis.

One such inflammatory messenger is tumor necrosis factor-alpha (TNF-alpha). It is found in increased concentration in the skin, blood, and joints of patients with psoriasis and psoriatic arthritis. TNF-alpha is normally present in the body at low levels. It plays a key role in mediating inflammation in the body and is an important messenger that helps cause many of the signs and symptoms of psoriasis and psoriatic arthritis. The continual release of TNF-alpha results in chronic inflammation with swelling and pain in the joints, and red, scaly, itchy lesions of psoriasis.

Blocking TNF-alpha can lead to significant improvement in

the skin and joints of patients with psoriasis and psoriatic arthritis.

Who Does It Affect?

Up to 15–30 percent of psoriasis sufferers will develop psoriatic arthritis. Psoriatic arthritis usually develops between the ages of 20 and 50, and is uncommon in children.

However, when the disease occurs in children, its development differs from that of adults. For example, in childhood, psoriatic arthritis affects females at three times the rate of males, whereas, in adulthood, women and men are affected equally. In addition, psoriatic arthritis develops before psoriasis in about 50 percent of children, compared to only 5 percent of adults. Almost 85 percent of adults with psoriatic arthritis develop psoriasis first.

Alice is a 55-year-old woman who has been married for thirty-five years, and has three daughters and five grandchildren. She is an enthusiastic, positive source of energy. I had the opportunity to meet her when her family doctor asked me to see her for scaly, red, raised areas of skin.

A year before I saw her, Alice's scalp began to itch and was scaly. After a few weeks of dealing with this symptom, she noticed patches of scaling, red skin developing on her legs. Her family doctor correctly diagnosed it as mild psoriasis, and she was started on a topical steroid cream and calcipotriol (Dovonex®, Daivonex®), a vitamin D–based cream. The topical creams had a modest effect in improving her symptoms; however, the affected areas would tend to recur as soon as the creams were stopped and, despite increasing strengths of topical steroids, new areas were appearing.

Alice was also developing two new problems. About eight months after Alice's first symptoms, she noticed that several of her nails were lifting from the skin. In addition, they were developing fine pits, as if a needle had been used to prick the surface of the nail, leaving multiple small defects in the nail plate. They were also becoming yellow, discolored, and thickened. Particularly troublesome was the fact that her right hip, both knees, and right ankle were becoming tender, swollen, and painful, as were her right index finger and the base of her left index finger. Alice was finding this arthritis crippling to the point where she could not pick up her grandchildren, and she was finding it difficult to sleep because of pain. Walking distances was becoming troublesome. She noted that the stiffness could improve sometimes throughout the day; however, it would tend to recur after a period of inactivity.

When I examined Alice, she had the classic symptoms of psoriasis in the scalp and elsewhere on the body. There were thick, red, well-demarcated patches and plaques involving approximately 15 percent of her body, particularly on the lower legs, arms, and scalp. Her fingernails had characteristic changes of psoriasis. She had obvious redness and swelling of the fingers, and these were painful and stiff on examination. Her fourth left toe had a characteristic change of psoriatic arthritis as there was diffuse swelling of the toe, and the skin was shiny and tight.

Given that she had extensive psoriasis and psoriatic arthritis, I explained to Alice that she would need a medication, taken orally or by injection, that would treat both of these conditions. Before starting this, we did some initial blood work, which revealed that she had a very mild anemia; tests for the rheumatoid factor and antinuclear antibody were both negative. I also ordered some X-rays of her joints and referred her to a rheumatologist for assessment and management of her painful joints. Given the extent of her psoriasis, we elected to start her on methotrexate (Rheumatrex®) (15 milligrams), by mouth, once weekly.

When I saw her again three months later, Alice had had an excellent response to the methotrexate with clearing of almost all of her psoriasis. By this time, she had seen the rheumatologist, who had agreed that methotrexate was an appropriate choice for her psoriatic arthritis. Her joint symptoms were slower to improve, but she was making definite progress, with a reduction in the swelling and stiffness. Alice was extremely happy with her progress and was encouraged by the fact that her activities had resumed to almost normal levels.

What Are the Signs and Symptoms of Psoriatic Arthritis?

Psoriatic arthritis can develop gradually and in its mildest form may produce minimal discomfort in those affected. In others, psoriatic arthritis may be severe and, if untreated, patients may become disabled with swollen, deformed joints.

Psoriatic arthritis can produce several symptoms:
- swelling and tenderness of joints
- stiffness and decreased ability to move joints fully
- pain and stiffness that is worse in the morning or with rest
- raised, scaly, red skin lesions may occur
- nail changes are very common, particularly if arthritis involves the joints at the ends of the fingers and toes
- redness and tenderness of the eye

Which Joints Can Be Affected?

Psoriatic arthritis can affect one or many joints, and will occur in certain patterns. To determine the pattern or different locations of joints affected, it is important to know:
- How many joints are affected? Is only a single joint affected (monoarthritis)? Are a few joints affected (oligoarthritis)? Or are multiple joints affected (polyarthritis)?

Finger Joints Commonly Affected by Psoriatic Arthritis

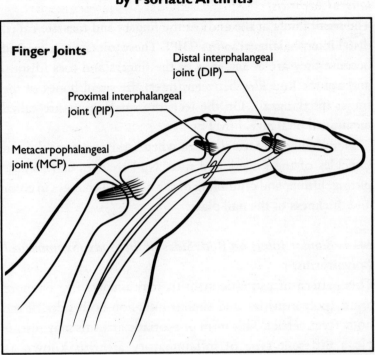

Finger Joints

Distal interphalangeal joint (DIP)

Proximal interphalangeal joint (PIP)

Metacarpophalangeal joint (MCP)

- Are the joints affected symmetrically (similar joints on both sides of the body)? For example, are the small joints of the right and left hands and feet affected? Or are the joints affected in an asymmetrical way (different joints involved on opposite sides of the body)?
- Is the joint involved causing deformity or mutilation?

More than thirty years ago, Dr. Moll and Dr. Wright described five clinical patterns of psoriatic arthritis, in which they explained the specific joints that were affected in different groups of patients:

End Knuckles of the Fingers and Toes (Distal Interphalangeal Arthritis)

The small joints at the ends of the fingers and toes are called distal interphalangeal joints (DIP). These joints are so named because they are at the ends of the fingers and toes (distal), and are the knuckles between (inter) the small bones of the finger (phalangeal). On the feet, the small joints are called metatarsal phalangeal (MTP).

Nail changes are usually seen when arthritis affects the end knuckles of the fingers and toes. Nail changes can include pitting, lifting, and crumbling of the nail, and changes in color and thickness of the nail plate.

Many Similar Joints on Both Sides of the Body (Symmetrical Polyarthritis)

This pattern of psoriatic arthritis may involve five or more joints (polyarthritis), and similar joints on both sides of the body (symmetric). This form of psoriatic arthritis may resemble a different type of inflammatory arthritis known as rheumatoid arthritis.

One or Only a Few Joints in an Asymmetrical Pattern (Mono or Asymmetrical Oligoarthritis)

Four or fewer joints are affected, usually in an asymmetrical pattern. This is the most common form of psoriatic arthritis and occurs in about 70 percent of all cases. For example, a large joint such as a knee may be involved with one or two small joints of the finger (DIP) or toe (MTP).

Spinal Involvement

This pattern of psoriatic arthritis involves the spine. The low back is most frequently affected.

Arthritis Mutilans

This is a severe form of psoriatic arthritis, which can be extremely disabling. As the name suggests, this form of arthritis can cause destruction and mutilation (mutilans) of the small joints of the fingers and toes. The fingers may appear swollen and sausage-like. Fortunately, this is a rare form occurring in fewer than 1 percent of all psoriatic arthritis cases.

These patterns can help in diagnosing psoriatic arthritis when the arthritis first develops. Over time, an increasing number of joints can become involved, and the pattern of involvement could change.

Are Tissues and Tendons Involved?

In addition to these distinctive patterns of joints, there are other unique features of psoriatic arthritis. These include distinct changes in the tissues surrounding the joints, involvement of tendons, and back pain.

Tissue Swelling

Redness and swelling at the DIP joints is common. Instead of the inflammation being confined to the joints, it can extend to the surrounding tissue such as the tendons, ligaments, and bone. This can result in red, swollen, sausage-like toes or fingers. This sausage-like swelling is called dactylitis.

Tendinitis and Enthesitis

Tendinitis is inflammation of the tendon, while enthesitis refers to inflammation where the tendons attach to the bone. "Tennis elbow" or "heel spurs" are two common painful forms of inflammation at the insertion of a tendon to a bone that occur in people without psoriatic arthritis.

In psoriatic arthritis, tendinitis and enthesitis commonly

affect the Achilles tendon or the plantar fascia (heel of the foot). Both can be quite painful, limiting the ability to walk.

Back Pain

In psoriatic arthritis patients, back pain can be caused by inflammation of the spine or lower back (sacroiliac joints). The pain is typically worse in the morning or at night, often waking the patient. Pain and stiffness can improve with activity. Males are more commonly affected than females.

These features may appear alone or in combination, and the characteristics may change over time. Signs and symptoms may vary from patient to patient.

Can Psoriatic Arthritis Affect Any Other Parts of the Body?

In addition to the skin and joints, psoriatic arthritis can affect the eye, urethra, heart, and bowel.

Eye

Up to one-third of patients may have inflammation of the eye, involving the white part of the eye (conjunctivitis) or the pigmented part of the eye (iritis).

Heart

An enlargement (or dilation) of one of the major arteries leading from the heart (aorta) may occur.

Urethra

The urethra is a narrow tube that empties the bladder. Urethritis is an inflammation of the urethra.

What Is the Relationship between the Severity of Psoriasis and Psoriatic Arthritis?

There is no direct, consistent relationship between the severity of the joint and skin diseases. In the past, it was believed that patients with extensive, severe psoriasis would be more likely to have arthritis. However, several recent studies have failed to find such a link either between the extent or the amount of skin disease and joint severity. One exception involves the frequent association of nail abnormalities in patients with involvement of the joints at the ends of the finger or toes.

Many will develop skin lesions before the development or diagnosis of joint disease. Approximately 10–15 percent of affected adults with psoriatic arthritis can present with joint disease first, without the presence of psoriasis skin lesions.

How Is Psoriatic Arthritis Diagnosed?

Helpful clues in the diagnosis of psoriatic arthritis include:
- psoriasis skin lesions (well-defined, red, scaling plaques with silvery scale)
- nail changes (pitting, lifting of the nail plate, yellow discoloration)
- asymmetric joint pain and swelling
- swollen fingers and toes (dactylitis)
- redness and swelling at end knuckles (DIPs) or middle knuckles (PIPs)
- enthesitis (inflammation and tenderness where a tendon attaches to the bone); Achilles tendon and heel are very common sites
- back pain
- joint stiffness in the morning

In general, a diagnosis of psoriatic arthritis is made on the basis of four features:
- medical history
- physical examination of joints
- laboratory and blood tests
- X-rays

Medical History

Since most patients with psoriatic arthritis will initially have psoriasis lesions, a medical history and physical examination are both very important in diagnosing psoriatic arthritis.

Your doctor might ask the questions in the chart on page 51 in order to help establish a diagnosis of psoriatic arthritis.

Physical Examination

In a person presenting with swollen, tender joints, an examination of the skin for typical lesions of psoriasis and nail changes can indicate the possibility of psoriatic arthritis. In addition to the skin exam, your doctor may make other assessments, such as taking your blood pressure, and listening to and examining your heart, lungs, and abdomen.

Your doctor will need to carefully examine your joints to look for changes in the joints, and identify the number of joints

---

Report Joint Symptoms to Your Doctor

Remember to discuss any joint symptoms with your family doctor and/or dermatologist. He or she will help determine whether you have psoriatic arthritis and might subsequently refer you to a rheumatologist.

---

affected. Many dermatologists refer patients to a rheumatologist for detailed examination of the joints and further testing.

Your doctor will look at, feel, and move your joints to assess the problem, and determine both the number of joints and the extent to which they are affected. Clues that suggest psoriatic arthritis include:

- the presence of hot, red joints
- sausage-like fingers and toes (dactylitis)

Questions Your Doctor May Ask	Why This Is Important
Does anyone else in your family have psoriatic arthritis?	Genetics, or inheritance, can play a role in the development of psoriatic arthritis.
Do you have pain and stiffness in your joints during the night? On awakening in the morning?	Inflammatory arthritis often presents with pain and stiffness in joints that are worse with rest and improved with activity.
How long does the pain and stiffness last?	Pain and stiffness that last about an hour may indicate inflammatory arthritis.
Do you have pain in your heel or Achilles tendon? Do you have tennis elbow?	Inflammation at the connection between the tendons and bones is known as enthesitis, and it is an important finding in psoriatic arthritis. Enthesitis may be noted as pain in the heel, Achilles tendon or in the elbow.
Do you have roughness, pitting or lifting of your nails?	Changes in your nails are highly associated with psoriatic arthritis.
Do you have any irritation in your eyes? Irritation passing urine?	Psoriatic arthritis can be associated with inflammation in sites other than your joints, such as your eyes (conjunctivitis, iritis), urethra (urethritis) and mucous membranes.
How is your energy?	Fatigue can be a major problem for some patients with psoriatic arthritis.

- different joints on opposite sides of the body (asymmetrical) are affected
- distal interphalangeal (DIP) joints are affected

Feeling the joints gives important information about the presence of warmth, swelling, and a grinding sensation known as crepitus.

Warmth in a joint can indicate inflammation, which is found in psoriatic arthritis as well as several other types of arthritis. Swelling in a joint can be due to several causes, e.g., thickening of the lining in the joints (known as synovium) or bony overgrowth. Crepitus refers to the sensation of crunching or grinding in a joint, which you can feel if your hand is placed over the joint while it is in motion.

Your doctor might feel your joints to determine whether you have pain when pressure is applied. In addition, inflammation at those sites where the tendon inserts into the bone is characteristic of psoriatic arthritis.

Finally, your doctor might try to move your joints through a range of movement, to see if they are normal. Those with deformities from psoriatic arthritis could have a limited range of movement. Your doctor will also evaluate the ability and strength of your grip.

Laboratory and Blood Tests

There is no single laboratory test that diagnoses psoriatic arthritis. Certain laboratory tests are usually performed to determine if there could be another cause for the arthritis. There are two important blood tests, including the rheumatoid factor and the antinuclear antibody (ANA).

The first test was described earlier; the second test excludes the presence of systemic lupus erythematosus (lupus). Antinuclear antibody is found in about 95 percent of people with lupus, but rarely in psoriatic arthritis. Because lupus symptoms are similar to those of psoriatic arthritis, a negative antinuclear test can help rule out lupus.

Your doctor could also order other blood tests to monitor the progress of your disease, rather than for diagnostic purposes. For example, an erythrocyte sedimentation rate (ESR) is a nonspecific test that can reflect the degree of joint inflammation.

Another test is a complete blood count (CBC), which is exactly that—a count of all the cells of the blood: red blood cells, white blood cells, and platelets. Red blood cells are important (they carry oxygen from the lungs to the rest of the body), and their levels can be reduced in those with psoriatic arthritis or other types of inflammatory arthritis. A decrease in the level of red blood cells is called anemia.

Joint Aspiration

A joint aspiration involves using a syringe to take fluid from a swollen joint. Examining the fluid for white blood cells, infection, or crystals found in other causes of arthritis can be very important for establishing the correct diagnosis.

X-rays

X-rays are helpful in making a correct diagnosis of psoriatic arthritis, and in evaluating the extent and severity of the arthritis. Sometimes people with psoriatic arthritis have little or no joint pain, so joint destruction can go unnoticed. An X-ray can show specific changes that help distinguish psoriatic arthritis from other types of arthritis. In addition, an X-ray can determine the extent of the damage to the joints and provide a baseline with which to compare later X-rays. The areas typically involved are the end and middle knuckle joints, the spine, the lower back at the base of the spine (sacroiliac joints), and at the site of tendon or ligament insertions to bone (entheses). If psoriasis is evident or psoriatic arthritis is suspected, X-rays of the hands, wrists, feet, and sacroiliac joints may be taken. Other areas can be X-rayed, depending on the patient's symptoms.

How Is Psoriatic Arthritis Treated?

Treatment includes managing both arthritis and skin lesions, when both are present, and will depend on the severity of the psoriasis and psoriatic arthritis. In many cases, the treatments are complementary, that is, if a dermatologist is treating your skin lesions with a systemic agent such as methotrexate or etanercept (Enbrel®) (Chapter 10), this treatment could also help your psoriatic arthritis. In many cases, patients with psoriatic arthritis will be referred to a rheumatologist. In most cases, your doctors (dermatologist, rheumatologist, family physician) will work together to help find the best treatment.

The dermatologist usually continues to follow your treatments and provide guidance for the care of your skin. The treatment of psoriasis is discussed in detail in chapters 8–12.

Treatments for psoriatic arthritis include the following:

Nonsteroidal Anti-inflammatory Drugs (NSAIDs)
- slow-acting anti-rheumatic drugs (SAARDs)/disease-modifying anti-rheumatic drugs (DMARDs)
- methotrexate
- cyclosporine
- antimalarials
- gold
- penicillamine (Cuprimine®, Depen®)
- sulfasalazine (Azulfidine®)

Biologic Agents
- etanercept (Enbrel®)
- infliximab (Remicade®)
- adalimumab (Humira®)

Experimental Biologic Agents
- alefacept (Amevive®)
- ustekinumab (Stelera®)

Nonsteroidal Anti-inflammatory Drugs (NSAIDs)
NSAIDs are anti-inflammatory drugs that help reduce pain and inflammation in mild psoriatic arthritis. NSAIDs also help control morning stiffness, which improves a patient's range of motion. NSAIDs have been reported to cause psoriasis flare-ups in some individuals, although this is an infrequent occurrence. There are a large number of NSAIDs available, but none is superior in terms of reducing inflammation.

Slow-Acting Antirheumatic Drugs (SAARDs)
As the name suggests, slow-acting antirheumatic drugs
(SAARDs) take weeks or months to show significant benefit
in most patients. This group is also called disease-modifying
anti-rheumatic drugs (DMARDs).

Methotrexate
Methotrexate is recognized as being highly effective in psoriasis and psoriatic arthritis. In the past, methotrexate has been
a preferred drug if patients have psoriasis and psoriatic arthritis because it has therapeutic benefits for both diseases. It can
be taken orally or by injection into the muscle. Potential side
effects include inflammation of the liver (hepatitis), scarring
of the liver (cirrhosis), and an increased risk for infection;
methotrexate is unsafe during pregnancy. Methotrexate is discussed in further detail in Chapter 10.

Cyclosporine
Cyclosporine is effective in treating psoriatic arthritis, although
it has a number of serious side effects, including high blood
pressure (hypertension) and damage to the kidney.
Cyclosporine is reviewed in detail in Chapter 11.

Antimalarials
Antimalarials are drugs originally developed for use against
malaria. Antimalarials such as chloroquine (Aralen®) and
hydroxychloroquine (Plaquenil®) have been used to treat psoriatic arthritis with modest success in limited studies. While
the safety profile is relatively good, certain patients report
worsening of their psoriasis when taking antimalarials.

Gold
Gold can be taken orally or by injection into the muscle.

Intramuscular injections are believed to be more effective than oral treatments. Although gold works for some patients, it does not prevent psoriatic arthritis from progressing. Gold can also take a long time before it begins to work. Common side effects of gold include a sore mouth, possibly with ulcers; itchy skin or widespread rash; and a reduction in certain components of the blood (platelets). If platelet levels drop, easy bruising or bleeding can occur at sites of minor trauma.

Penicillamine (Cuprimine®)
Penicillamine provides some benefit, but its slow onset of action and side effects have limited its use in the treatment of psoriatic arthritis. Common side effects of penicillamine include nausea, and an unusual metallic taste and sores in the mouth. Less commonly, increased risk of bleeding due to the drop in platelet levels, and protein in the urine can be seen.

Sulfasalazine
Sulfasalazine may be used alone or in combination with other medications. Sulfasalazine has only limited effectiveness when used alone to treat psoriatic arthritis and is not well tolerated by many patients. Common side effects of sulfasalazine include abdominal discomfort, nausea, decreased appetite, and headache. Less commonly, the liver may be inflamed (hepatitis), and white blood cell and platelet counts may drop. This can result in an increased susceptibility to infection (due to decreased white blood cells) and bleeding (due to decreased platelets).

Biologic Agents
A new type of medication being studied and used for the treatment of psoriasis and psoriatic arthritis is called a biologic agent because of the way they are synthesized and the fact that they are proteins. The significant advances in understanding

the causes of psoriasis and psoriatic arthritis have resulted in the development of this new class of medications. The biologic drugs target the abnormality in the immune system to modify the biology of the person with psoriasis or psoriatic arthritis back to normal. Biologic agents are reviewed in detail in Chapter 12.

As discussed, tumor necrosis factor-alpha (TNF-alpha) is one of many inflammatory messengers that can cause the tender, swollen joints of psoriatic arthritis and the red, scaly, raised areas of skin in psoriasis. TNF-alpha is increased in the skin and joints of patients with psoriasis and psoriatic arthritis. When TNF-alpha is increased, it causes a number of changes in the blood vessels, skin, and joints, which can result in inflammation in the skin and joints. Reducing the activated T-cells that cause the release of TNF-alpha or blocking this inflammatory messenger can reduce inflammation (redness and swelling) of the joints and improve the skin lesions of psoriasis.

Currently, three biologic agents that block TNF-alpha are being used in psoriatic arthritis: infliximab, etanercept, and adalimumab. These agents are able to neutralize the undesirable inflammatory effects by controlling the amount of TNF-alpha in the skin and joints.

In addition, alefacept, a biologic agent that can reduce the number of T-cells that cause the release of TNF-alpha, has been recently studied in psoriatic arthritis and found to be effective. These two biologic agents are explained in more detail in Chapter 12. Here, I will briefly outline the experience with these agents in psoriatic arthritis.

Infliximab
- Infliximab targets and blocks the inflammatory messenger TNF-alpha by binding to it.

- Infliximab acts like a sponge to take TNF-alpha out of circulation.
- The drug is given by intravenous infusion over approximately a two-hour period.
- Infliximab has also been used to treat rheumatoid arthritis and Crohn's disease (an inflammatory disease of the bowel).
- Infliximab has undergone recent clinical testing in psoriatic arthritis, but is not yet approved in Canada for psoriatic arthritis.
- A clinical study, the Infliximab Multinational Psoriatic Arthritis Controlled Trial (IMPACT), recently reported that about 70 percent of patients had an improvement as measured by a clinical score (ACR-20), over a sixteen-week study. In addition, 67 percent had an excellent improvement in the psoriasis.

Etanercept

- Etanercept targets and blocks the inflammatory messenger TNF-alpha in a different way than infliximab.
- Etanercept is a fully human receptor that circulates in the blood and acts like a sponge to take TNF-alpha out of circulation. Etanercept binds to TNF-alpha, preventing TNF-alpha from both binding to the inflammatory cell and sending it a faulty message. By blocking this faulty message, inflammation is reduced.
- Etanercept is self-administered by patients in one of two ways:
  1. Once weekly: Two injections under the skin (subcutaneous) of 25 milligrams each on the same day.
  2. Twice weekly: One injection under the skin (subcutaneous) of 25 milligrams three to four days apart.
- Etanercept has been extensively studied in psoriatic arthritis in well-designed, randomized, controlled trials.

- In one recent study, etanercept was given to 205 patients with psoriatic arthritis. Patients were given one injection (25 milligrams) of etanercept or placebo under the skin (subcutaneous), twice weekly over twenty-four weeks. A rapid and significant improvement was reported in 59 percent of patients receiving etanercept using the measured score (ACR-20). Significant improvements in skin lesions were also reported by 57 percent of patients.
- Etanercept has been studied alone and in combination with other treatments such as methotrexate and other NSAIDs.
- Etanercept is currently approved in the United States and Canada for the treatment of psoriatic arthritis.

Adalimumab
- Adalimumab blocks tumor necrosis factor-alpha (TNF-alpha) by binding to it.
- Adalimumab is administered as an injection every other week.
- Adalimumab works quickly (many patients notice an improvement within the first month).
- Studies have shown an excellent improvement in psoriasis and psoriatic arthritis.
- Adalimumab has also been used in combination with other types of treatment, such as methotrexate, NSAIDs, or SAARDs in the treatment of psoriatic arthritis.
- The most common side effects include reaction at the injection site, cold, headache, and flu-like symptoms.

Alefacept
- Alefacept blocks the activation of T-cells and reduces the number of activated T-cells that contribute to the release of inflammatory mediators.
- It is administered by intramuscular injection.

- Alefacept has undergone recent clinical trial evaluation in psoriatic arthritis, but is not yet approved for use in psoriatic arthritis in Canada. A recent clinical study using alefacept and methotrexate resulted in significant improvement in patients with psoriatic arthritis.

Ustekinumab (Stelera)

- Ustekinumab targets and blocks chemical messengers (cytokines), interleukin-12, and interleukin-23.
- Ustekinumab has been used in a recent study in patients with psoriatic arthritis and has been found to improve psoriatic arthritis.
- Clinical trials are currently ongoing to establish the effectiveness of this medication in the treatment of psoriatic arthritis.

Nonmedical Treatments

In addition to oral or injectable medications, there are a number of nonmedical, physical, and surgical treatments for psoriatic arthritis. The management of psoriatic arthritis is a team approach. In addition to your family doctor, dermatologist, and rheumatologist, you may work with a physiotherapist or occupational therapist.

Physiotherapy

Physiotherapists are university-trained health care workers who try to help people achieve their highest level of physical function. Physiotherapists can develop and implement personalized programs that can:

- increase mobility and improve endurance
- restore and increase range of motion in joints
- control pain

- educate patients about their condition and pain-control techniques

Exercise

Moderate to low-impact exercise can:
- maintain and improve joint range of motion
- reduce weight and pressure on joints
- improve aerobic capacity and cardiovascular fitness
- relieve joint stiffness and pain
- improve strength

Hydrotherapy/Aquatherapy

Aquatherapy or water therapy is a series of exercises performed in the pool. Exercises performed in the water are low impact, and therefore easier on painful, swollen joints.

Hot or Cold Therapy

Hot wraps with a towel or hot pack can relieve painful muscle soreness and joint pain. Cold therapy can reduce swelling and tenderness of psoriatic arthritis. A cheap and effective cold pack is a bag of frozen vegetables. It can be easily molded to affected joints, and the cold can help reduce the swelling and pain of psoriatic arthritis.

Occupational Therapy

Occupational therapists help provide assistance in activity and tasks of daily life in patients with psoriatic arthritis. As the name implies, occupational therapists may work with patients to facilitate their occupations, including self-care, leisure, tasks of daily life, and workplace activities.

Occupational therapists are able to assist people in continuing to perform activities of importance to them. For example, a patient with arthritis mutilans may have difficulty grasping objects or opening a jar of food. Occupational therapists can help provide solutions with innovative tools to assist in activities and maintain such abilities. If you have severe psoriatic arthritis with deformed joints, you can learn new and different ways to complete daily tasks.

Surgery

Given the many medical and physical treatments discussed above, most people with psoriatic arthritis will never need surgery. Patients with severely damaged and deformed joints may require surgical procedures such as:

- *Synovectomy:* This is a surgical procedure involving removal of all or a portion of the lining of the joint (synovial membrane) or diseased portion of the joint to improve function.
- *Arthropathy or joint-replacement surgery:* This involves replacing natural joints with an artificial joint.

Your Health Care Team

The overall management of psoriasis and psoriatic arthritis is a team effort, often including a dermatologist, rheumatologist, family physician, and other health care specialists like physiotherapists and occupational therapists. Educating the patient about psoriatic arthritis is an important responsibility for the team. The patient should be informed that psoriatic arthritis is a long-term, persistent inflammatory disease, and that steady therapy is required. A combination of drugs and rehabilitation methods may be needed for therapy. The patient's responsibility involves maintaining a healthy lifestyle by exercising to preserve or improve joint mobility. The patient should also follow treatment steps accordingly.

SIX

Psoriasis in Children

Psoriasis, unlike eczema, is less common in childhood. The exact prevalence in childhood is not well established, and there is some variation in reports and studies. In general, up to one-third of patients with psoriasis report the onset of disease before the age of 20. One large study found that in 12 percent of adult patients, the onset occurred before the age of 10, and in 25 percent, between the ages of 10 and 19. A recent Australian study reported the largest number of children with psoriasis ever, and approximately one-quarter of them developed the disease before the age of 2.

When psoriasis occurs in childhood, the lesions are usually plaques with raised, red scaly areas, but can be thinner and less scaly than their adult counterparts. In addition, childhood psoriasis is reported to be itchier (pruritic) than in adults.

Psoriasis in children is frequently precipitated by infection, and guttate psoriasis is not uncommon (see Chapter 1). This type of psoriasis presents with multiple scaling and raised areas of skin that develop rapidly on the body; however, it can resolve completely with no recurrence.

The good news is that psoriasis, in general, will not affect your child's health, growth, or development. With the proper treatment, especially for the majority of children with mild disease, this condition can be well controlled and will have little impact on their emotional and physical health. In children with more severe, extensive, and chronic or persistent forms of psoriasis, it is important to realize that there are many new treatments being investigated, and that the future for effective control of psoriasis has never been brighter.

What Does Psoriasis Look Like in Children?

Psoriasis can begin at or shortly after birth, but in most children it usually does not occur until school age. A family history of the disorder is quite common. When present in babies or infants, it commonly starts in the diaper area (napkin psoriasis) and can spread elsewhere on the body. In children, psoriasis can develop as small, flat, or raised, red, discrete areas that develop a thick, silvery scale. These small areas can join to form raised, thick, scaling plaques with a sharp border separating involved and uninvolved skin. Common sites involved include the scalp, ears, elbows, knees, buttock crease, genitals, and nails. The most common form of psoriasis in children is chronic plaque-type psoriasis, with raised, thick, scaling areas. Psoriatic arthritis is quite rare in children.

In up to one-third of cases in children, the initial development of psoriasis can involve multiple, small, teardrop-shaped, scaling, raised lesions, known as guttate psoriasis (see Chapter 1). Children might experience an outbreak of guttate psoriasis following a cold (upper respiratory infection), most commonly a bacterial infection of the throat (streptococcal pharyngitis or strep throat). Occasionally, a bacterial infection (streptococcal) of the rectum can lead to a flare-up of guttate psoriasis. Also, if the child is prone to tonsillitis, psoriasis could recur with future cases of tonsillitis. Guttate psoriasis most commonly affects the back, abdomen, arms, and legs. While a child might have a fever with a bacterial infection, it is unusual for children to have a fever with psoriasis.

In children as in adults, psoriasis can develop at the site of an injury (Koebner phenomenon). Psoriasis can occur in a straight line along a scratch or appear after abrasions, cuts, or insect bites. This information can be a helpful clue in diagnosing psoriasis.

Scalp involvement is very common in children. Thick, scaling, raised lesions can involve either localized areas of the scalp, such as behind the ears and/or along the hairline, or the entire scalp. This can result in the shedding of white scales from the scalp, commonly mistaken for dandruff.

The genitals are also frequently affected in children, particularly babies. The penis, groin, buttock crease, and labia are common sites of involvement. The fingernails and toenails might also be involved. The nails may become pitted or rough, and the distal part of the nail can become quite thick and crumbly. Lifting of the nail from the surrounding skin can also occur (onycholysis). Occasionally in children, all twenty nails may be involved.

Other forms of psoriasis seen in adults, such as erythrodermic and pustular psoriasis, are less common in childhood (see Chapter 2).

With treatment, psoriasis can be controlled effectively in children.

Devon is an active, happy, 2-year-old toddler who was referred to me by her family doctor because of a recurrent diaper rash. The rash had started on her buttocks a year earlier after an episode of diarrhea. Subsequently, she developed a red, scaly rash, which healed after treatment with a mild topical steroid cream. However, it recurred in the genital area and had been persistent for the past four to five months. There is a family history of psoriasis involving Devon's father and grandfather. Her father has more extensive involvement on the arms and legs, which has been ongoing for more than ten years, with a history of psoriatic arthritis.

Recently, Devon also developed a red scaly area on the left eyelid; her parents wondered if there was any relationship to the diaper rash and were concerned about the potential for scarring. They are worried—as Devon tends to scratch these areas frequently—that this condition could worsen when she is older. At this point, they were using only zinc oxide cream to treat the areas in the diaper region.

Devon is an otherwise completely healthy girl who is very active and has had normal growth and development. She likes to play with her older sister, who is 3 1/2 years old, and there has been no limitation, because of this condition, on her activities.

When I examined Devon, I detected very localized disease with only the presence of redness and minimal scaling on the genitals and the lower abdomen, as well as a very small amount of scaling and redness on the left upper eyelid.

I explained to Devon's parents that the rash in the diaper area and on the eyelid was childhood psoriasis, and that the involvement of the diaper area is often seen in young children. I started Devon on treatment with hydrocortisone 1 percent ointment rather than the cream as an ointment is more moisturizing. In addition, I prescribed one of the newer nonsteroidal treatments, pimecrolimus 1 percent cream, for use on the face and also, as needed, for the genital area. Nonsteroidal therapies can avoid the side effects of steroids in the skin when used over longer periods. They are currently under investigation for treatment of psoriasis in delicate skin. It is important, however, to recognize that topical steroids can be used quite safely for shorter periods in delicate areas or on other body areas for longer periods.

Devon completely cleared with this treatment and subsequently has had only occasional mild involvement in these areas.

What Else Can Look Like Psoriasis in Children?

Several other conditions can resemble psoriasis in children, and might be mistaken for psoriasis.

Pityriasis Rosea

- Pityriasis rosea is a skin rash that occurs most commonly in people aged 10–35.
- Pityriasis rosea can follow a cold (upper respiratory infection), much like guttate psoriasis, and may be confused with this type of psoriasis.
- The condition may begin as a single, large, scaling, pink patch (larger than 3/8 inch/1 centimeter, flat) on the chest or back.
- About a week or two later, multiple, flat, scaling, pink-red patches occur on the chest, back, upper arms, and legs.
- The face and scalp are seldom involved, whereas in psoriasis the scalp is frequently involved.
- The rash usually fades over about eight weeks.

Seborrheic Dermatitis

- Seborrheic dermatitis is a common skin disorder that is red, scaly, and occasionally itchy.
- Scaling of the scalp appears yellow and is greasy in texture.
- It most commonly involves the scalp, sides of the nose, eyebrows, eyelids, and middle of the chest.

- It occurs most frequently in infancy when it is known as cradle cap. Cradle cap usually clears between 1 and 2 years of age.
- In some infants, seborrheic dermatitis may occur in the diaper area, where it may be confused with other types of diaper rashes, including psoriasis (napkin psoriasis).

Atopic Dermatitis/Eczema

- Eczema is a common chronic and recurring inflammation of the skin.
- About 90 percent of eczema cases begin in childhood, usually before the age of 5. In contrast, psoriasis tends to occur in older children and adults, and usually develops between the ages of 15 and 35.
- Scaling in atopic dermatitis is usually mild. Scaling in psoriasis can be severe.
- Asthma and hay fever can occur with eczema.
- Eczema affects approximately 10–20 percent of children.
- Eczema is very itchy and is often known as the "itch that rashes."
- The skin in eczema appears red and cracked (fissures), and it is often difficult to see a clear line between involved and uninvolved skin. In psoriasis, the skin is red, thick, with silvery-white scales and, less commonly, forms cracks (fissures). It is easy to see a clear line between involved and uninvolved skin.
- Children with eczema are prone to skin infections such as viral infections (warts, cold sore infection) and bacterial infections of the skin with yellow crusting.
- Eczema tends to present with different patterns (areas of involvement on the body) than psoriasis. In babies and infants, eczema involves the face and neck. In children and

adolescents, the inner crease of the arm, behind the knees, and the face are sites that are frequently involved.

• Psoriasis tends to involve areas of the body that are the opposite of eczema: the elbows, the front of the knees, and the scalp, and often spares the face.

Candida (Yeast) Infection

• Genital psoriasis can be confused with candida infections.
• Candida infections of the skin are caused by a type of yeast.
• Candida can occur anywhere on the body, but favors skin creases such as those under the breasts, armpits, and groin.
• A scraping of the skin can be examined under a microscope or sent to the laboratory for culture. This will help distinguish between candida (positive culture) and psoriasis (negative culture).

Treatments for Children

The treatment of psoriasis in children depends on the location, extent, and severity of the lesions. The treatment of psoriasis is dealt with in greater detail in Chapters 8–12. Children should be advised not to scratch or pick the areas involved as this can worsen the skin and lead to new areas of development.

Basic treatments include moisturizers and baths. Baths can be soothing, especially for itchy areas. Adding a bath oil or tar to the water can be helpful.

Topical Steroids

Topical steroids are very helpful and are frequently prescribed. Low- to mid-potency steroids may be used for short periods on the trunk, scalp, and extremities as instructed by your doctor. Medium- or high-potency steroids can also be used for short periods on the arms and body as instructed by your doctor.

Nonsteroidal Creams and Ointments

Calcipotriol

Calcipotriol (Dovonex®, Daivonex®) decreases redness and scaliness, but can cause burning in some children, particularly on sensitive areas, such as the face.

Anthralin

Anthralin (Psoriatec®) can be applied and left, or applied for a short period, then washed off. This is known as short contact anthralin therapy (SCAT). Application time is generally increased with subsequent applications until the psoriasis lesions have improved.

Coal Tar

There are different types of coal tar used to treat psoriasis-affected skin (shale, wood, coal, and crude coal tar). Crude coal tar is one of the oldest psoriasis treatment options available, although many children and parents dislike using tar because it may be messy, smelly, and irritating. However, coal tar can provide significant benefit for patients and is available in a topical form and a shampoo form for the treatment of scalp psoriasis.

Topical coal tar is available as a gel, cream, ointment, liquid, bath solution, or shampoo. Coal tar can stain white or blond hair, clothing, towels, and bedding. If you apply treatment before going to bed, use old pajamas and bedding. Coal tar can make the skin more sensitive to sunlight (photosensitizer), so be careful when exposing your skin to sunlight when you have it on and carefully follow your doctor's instructions.

Calcineurin Inhibitors

These are currently under investigation for psoriasis and may be helpful for face, groin, and genital areas. They are available in ointment (tacrolimus [Protopic®] 0.1 percent and 0.03 percent) or cream (pimecrolimus [Elide®] 1 percent) forms.

Calcineurin inhibitors can cause slight burning with initial application. This burning is mild and tends to last only a few minutes. The burning generally resolves completely after one to two weeks of repeated use.

Tazarotene
Tazarotene (Tazorac®) has been used to treat psoriasis, but can cause irritation. It is often necessary to use topical steroids in conjunction with tazarotene to reduce irritation.

Phototherapy
Phototherapy can be considered for older children who fail to respond to topical treatments (see Chapter 10).

Systemic Medications
Systemic agents such as methotrexate and cyclosporine are used only in children with severe psoriasis or psoriatic arthritis.

Biologics
Etanercept has been approved for children with certain types of arthritis (juvenile rheumatoid arthritis), and has been studied in children aged 4–17 (see Chapter 12).

Practical Tips for Treating Psoriasis in Babies and Infants
Remember, your child's psoriasis will not, generally, affect his or her general health, growth, and development. Itching is often more common in children with psoriasis; however, scratching can aggravate the skin and make the condition worse. Here are some practical tips:

- Keep your child's nails short and cover hands with cotton gloves as needed.
- Baths with oil or oatmeal added can be soothing.
- Bathe in lukewarm—not hot or cold—water.
- Regularly apply moisturizers, especially after bathing.
- Apply topical corticosteroids as prescribed by your doctor.
- Oral antihistamines may be recommended by your doctor and can help reduce the tendency to scratch. If your child scratches at night, the nighttime use of antihistamines can both reduce scratching and aid in sleeping. A doctor should be consulted before using antihistamines as overuse can result in excessive sedation.
- To treat the redness and scaling of psoriasis in children, your doctor might prescribe topical corticosteroids.

Kayla is a 10-year-old girl who has had psoriasis since she was approximately 5 years of age. Initially, her psoriasis began in a localized area on her left calf. In the past few years it has gradually and progressively become more widespread, now involving most areas of her body. When she came to see me, she complained that her skin was itchy, and she noted the psoriasis was involving her arms, back, legs, scalp, and, more recently, her face. There is a family history of psoriasis (her grandmother).

In the past, Kayla had tried a number of topical therapies, which had initially helped clear the scaly, red, raised areas and reduced the itching. More recently, the topical steroid creams have not been effective, even in increasing strengths. She had also tried topical tars, but had found these to be irritating to her skin. Because she had failed these topical treatments, she was prescribed ultraviolet light, three times weekly for the past two years, which had helped at first, but was no longer effective.

When I first met Kayla she was noticeably shy and withdrawn. Her father explained to me later that her psoriasis was having a significant impact on her self-image and confidence. She was becoming more withdrawn and was unwilling to engage in physical activities that exposed her skin. She had occasionally been teased at school by some of the other children.

When I examined Kayla's skin, approximately 70 percent of her body was covered with psoriasis, sparing only areas of her face and several areas on her trunk. Kayla was certainly one of the most severe cases of psoriasis that I had seen in a child. It was clear to me why many of the topical therapies she had tried were no longer working. In patients with extensive psoriasis like Kayla, topical therapies are usually neither practical—requiring considerable time and effort to apply to such widespread areas—nor effective. Typically we need to use phototherapy or consider systemic therapies (oral or injections) to obtain a response.

Another dermatologist had referred Kayla to me because the phototherapy was no longer effective, and we were conducting a clinical study for psoriasis in children. This study involved using a novel agent that worked by blocking a protein called tumor-necrosis factor (TNF). TNF is important in helping the immune system to function normally. In patients with psoriasis and psoriatic arthritis, however, TNF is increased and plays a key role in causing the thick, red, scaly skin and swollen joints of psoriasis and psoriatic arthritis. Our clinical study involved blocking TNF and had been proven highly effective in treating psoriasis and psoriatic arthritis in adults. I discussed the risks and benefits with Kayla and her parents, and they were very interested in proceeding with this study.

When I saw Kayla two weeks after starting the therapy, she was significantly better as approximately 50 percent of her lesions had cleared up; at two months after starting the therapy, she was virtually clear. What was most striking to me was not the improvement in her psoriasis, but the improvement in her outlook, mood, and personality. Where she had been withdrawn and shy, she became quite bubbly, was happy to be in the office, and readily engaged in conversation. Kayla wrote me a letter that she wanted to share with other children in the study so that it might help them cope with psoriasis. Kayla agreed to let me include it here (see sidebar below).

Kayla's Letter to Other Kids

My name is Kayla. I am on the study for psoriasis. I have to take two needles every Thursday. It hurts a bit, but if you hold onto something or say something over and over again, it takes your mind off of it. To people who are on the trial, I am glad that you have gotten this wonderful chance to be on the trial. Trust me because I know. I am on the real drug and let me tell you it is the best thing I have ever done in my life! Now when I wear a T-shirt, I am not wondering what people think of my arms. I can finally wear short skirts like my friends. I have started to swim in public places. To think of it, I haven't done that for more than four years, so you can imagine how happy I am to be in this study. Sometimes I want to say that's enough, I don't want to do it anymore, but I just tell myself why I am going through this and I never say enough. One reason is that I want to go to my prom and not have any psoriasis on my body, wear shorts to the mall and anywhere else that matters. I don't want my children and grandchildren to have to go through what I had to go through.

Managing Your Child's Psoriasis at School and at Home

Often the biggest challenge that children with psoriasis face is the reaction of their peers. Unfortunately, other children might tease your child because of the appearance of his or her skin. Therefore, it is important that you support your child, listen to his or her concerns, and teach him or her about the disease. If other children are persistently teasing, it might be helpful to meet with your child's teacher to discuss the condition. It is vital that teachers and students understand psoriasis is not contagious. You can discuss your child's condition with teachers at the beginning of the school year and follow up with them during the year. If necessary, you might discuss with the teacher how best to educate classmates about the condition.

Embarrassment about the appearance of psoriasis can cause low self-esteem, make your child self-conscious about his or her appearance, and could lead the child to avoid taking part in social or physical activities.

The National Psoriasis Foundation has a Web site with a section for children and teens that allows them to chat online with similarly affected kids, which helps them to both cope with their disease and feel less isolated. The American Academy of Dermatology has a summer camp (for children and teens) that enables kids to meet other children with skin disorders and to learn about and understand these diseases (see "Further Resources," page 188).

Here are some practical tips for treating and coping with psoriasis in older children and teens, and for discussing psoriasis with your child:

- Educate yourself and your child about the disease.
- Be direct and open about the condition.
- Reassure your child that feeling angry, sad, and frustrated is normal so she or he can learn to accept the disease and not let the condition have a negative impact.
- Help your child become comfortable talking about psoriasis, not only with you but also with doctors and others who can offer support.
- Emphasize that you can't give psoriasis to people by touching them or sitting next to them.
- Listen to your child's concerns.
- Indicate that there are good treatments to help control the condition and reduce itchiness.

- Assure your child that his or her general health will not be affected, and that the condition is not life-threatening.
- Comfort your child by explaining that she or he is not alone. Many other children have this condition.
- Your child can continue to do all activities (sports/hobbies) that other children do.
- Help your child understand that by following your doctor's routine to treat psoriasis, the condition can be kept under control.

SEVEN

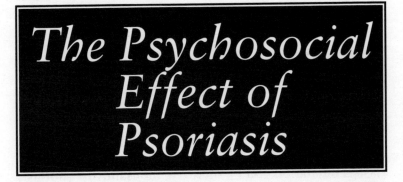

The Psychosocial Effect of Psoriasis

Psoriasis can have a significant impact on both your physical and mental health, resulting in impaired emotional and social well-being due to low self-esteem and possibly impaired functioning at work and in relationships.

Quality of Life

Psoriasis patients can experience many feelings about their diagnosis, including:

- a sense of shock
- confusion
- anger
- frustration
- great sadness
- depression

If not recognized and treated, these emotions can strain relationships, careers, and self-esteem. Ultimately, these pressures can have an extreme impact on a patient's quality of life.

Quality of life is measured by the impact of disease on a patient's lifestyle and emotional well-being and ability to participate in day-to-day activities, including:

- normal daily activities
- work activities
- relationships
- social life

Studies show that people with moderate to severe psoriasis experience a greater negative effect on their quality of life because of their disease. In the United States, the National Psoriasis Foundation (NPF) surveyed thousands of psoriasis patients from November 2001 to January 2002. The NPF found that of those patients with moderate to severe psoriasis, 77 percent felt the disease was a moderate to large problem in their lives. In addition, 26 percent said that because of their psoriasis they had to change or stop normal activities; 40 percent said they wear clothing that covers or hides their skin condition; and 36 percent said their psoriasis affects their ability to sleep.

Many times, those who don't suffer from psoriasis fail to understand the significant negative, physical, and emotional impact the disease can have on affected patients. Even doctors may not realize how this disease can negatively affect patients. In 1999, a survey was done of patients with different medical conditions, including psoriasis. These researchers measured the physical and mental impact of having these different diseases. They found that psoriasis patients experience among the greatest negative impacts on physical and mental well-being. The impact was so great that it exceeded that of high blood pressure (hypertension), diabetes, and even certain types of cancer.

Patients' quality of life is an important factor in treating the disease. One of the tools that researchers use to study the disease's effect on patients' lives is the Psoriasis Disability Index, a simple, disease-specific questionnaire containing fifteen questions, the answers to which are based on a patient's routine for the previous four weeks. The overall score reflects the degree of impact the patient has experienced during that time. A copy of the Psoriasis Disability Index questionnaire is included at the end of this chapter.

Dr. Stephen B. Perrott, a psoriasis patient who is a professor of psychology, wrote the next section. His unique experience and background is ideal for further explanation and discussion of the emotional, psychological, and physical impact of psoriasis. The purpose of this section is to educate you about the emotional and social effects that moderate to severe psoriasis can have, and what you can do about it as a person with psoriasis, a family member, or a friend.

Stephen's Story: A Personal Account

"It's gross." True enough. I have frequently thought of my moderate to severe psoriasis as being gross, not to mention embarrassing, painful, humiliating, time consuming, and depressing. However, for me to say my psoriasis is gross is one thing—for someone else to say it is wrenching. So, it is not hard to imagine how awful I felt about myself when my wife of more than twenty years made reference to my condition in this way in the dying days of our marriage. As much as people with psoriasis tell themselves so, and despite the reassurances of people who love us, it is not much of a leap from thinking that our psoriasis is gross to thinking that we are gross.

This is not to say that my wife did not have a point, or that my psoriasis did not have an impact on her life. After all, my constant shedding meant that I could never keep up with the flaky scales sprinkled across the hardwood floors, and it is not pleasant to wake up with bedsheets soiled with blood from cracked lesions. Let's face it; you have to look well inside a person before you can find much delight in cuddling up to someone covered in psoriasis plaque.

Walking the Road with Psoriasis

My experience with psoriasis started innocently enough in my mid-20s when my scalp became covered. At that point I remember thinking about the "heartbreak of psoriasis" and chuckling. After all, how tough could it be? Some extra money for special shampoo and a little unsightliness didn't seem to add up to "heartbreak." By my late 20s the psoriasis moved to my shins, and by my early 30s it had moved to my knees and elbows. Still, I was dealing only with spots, and it seemed that this unwelcome intruder would be kept at bay. I was wrong.

By the time I was 40 my psoriasis had left no significant area below my neck untouched. I am grateful that my face and chest are mostly clear. My arms, legs, back, and buttocks are write-offs. Most recently, scaling has appeared on the back of my hands, an area previously untouched except for the weird-looking fingernails that I keep trimmed as close to the skin as possible. Psoriasis's kissing cousin—psoriatic arthritis—also appeared at age 40, adding very sharp pain to the existing lower-level pain and itching that has affected my skin for 20 years.

As the psoriasis on my body became increasingly worse, my scalp cleared and has remained mostly clear to the present. Trust me, the trade-off has not been worth it. Most readers with serious psoriasis will not be surprised to hear about the relief to my scalp. This is a mysterious disease that moves around without much rhyme or reason. One day you can be excited that a particularly nasty patch disappears almost overnight and disappointed the next day when a previously clear area sprouts a new lesion. This unpredictability adds an additional component of stress to the psoriasis experience. Most human beings strive for predictability (consistency) in their lives and often do well when facing adverse experiences once a degree of control is established. Psoriasis is an intruder that mocks predictability and control.

As a chronic disease, psoriasis remains stubborn in the face of treatment. Treatment has provided me with a degree of comfort and some manageability, but no indication that I will ever beat the disease. Within the realm of treatment I have been fortunate. My dermatologist is not only a superb doctor, but also a truly decent person whose compassion and attentiveness have provided me with an immeasurable degree of psychological support. I am also fortunate to live in an urban center that provides me with ready access to the best treatment resources available.

So, have I tried to fight back? Sure. It all started with topical ointments that, from the beginning, had only limited success. Although time consuming and greasy on my clothes, the ointments would have been a small price to pay had they only worked. The second step included PUVA (psoralen plus ultraviolet-A) and UVB (ultraviolet-B) treatments. At this point treatment moved past the annoying to the truly disruptive level. Hundreds of trips and hundreds of hours under the lights initially helped considerably, but I was soon faced with the law of diminishing returns. Though light treatments are manageable, they do present challenges. I was usually left with a feeling of prickliness, and on several occasions found myself burned after pressuring nurses to give me more light than they thought advisable. PUVA also presented a particularly nasty surprise early on: the infamous "PUVA itch" from UVA (ultraviolet-A) light. Anyone who has experienced this knows that "itch" doesn't quite cover the experience. I once suffered a very long weekend with pain that almost drove me to the emergency room. This problem was knocked out with an anticonvulsant drug, another modification added to my already complicated treatment protocol.

By this point, I had turned into a sun worshipper from someone who had previously found that time in the sun constituted a waste of time (to say nothing of being potentially dangerous). Several summers provided an uplift in spirit as a couple of days in the sun would almost completely clear my skin. However, consecutive days in the warm sun are rare occurrences in Nova Scotia and eventually even those exposures were met with diminished returns.

So, I was onto methotrexate (Rheumatrex®) treatment, a step I embarked upon only after careful consultation with my dermatologist. Again, this initially worked well, but was not without side effects. Although I never became grossly ill with this anticancer drug, the day following my weekly treatment was usually accompanied by low-level nausea. Eventually, this resulted in a kind of conditioned nausea such that I would begin feeling ill before taking the tablets and often found myself gagging when swallowing them (readers should note that many people are successful in taking low-level doses of methotrexate without the nausea I experienced).

Ultimately, I again met with diminishing returns, necessitating an increased dose. As my dermatologist and I began considering options after blood tests gave rise to concern about liver function, a choice was made for us. I developed a nasty case of mucositis, an infection of the interior of the mouth that resulted from my lowered immune response. My run with methotrexate ceased.

Well, this seemed like the end of the road for treatment, and I resigned myself to managing the disease as best as I could. And, despite what I have already said, this was not the most crushing realization life had provided. Life is good, and psoriasis is not so debilitating that I would allow it to steal my entire quality of life. I add this in case the portrait I have painted so far leaves readers with less severe conditions fearing bleak futures. This is simply not the case, a feeling with which I suspect that others with even more severe conditions than mine would agree. I concluded that ongoing management would allow me to continue with a full life, and to this premise I added the strong message that I should accept the things I cannot change and realize that others face much worse conditions.

Accepting the things we cannot control does not equal giving up. During the last year much media attention has focused on the optimistic view that scientists and dermatologists are generating a number of emerging experimental treatments. When my dermatologist asked if I wanted to be involved in a clinical test of one of these treatments, I jumped at the chance. I am currently in the middle of a "double-blind" trial that involves weekly injections. The agent injected is called alefacept (Amevive®) which hopefully will respond with a methotrexate-like effect while bypassing the nasty nausea. Most importantly, this biological agent battles the T-cells responsible for the rapid growth of the epidermis without challenging the rest of the immune system (such as is the case with methotrexate). The double-blind strategy is an experimental method whereby some patients are injected with alprocet and others get a placebo (in this case a saline solution). It is too early yet to determine whether it is working for me or even if I am getting the real agent (neither I nor the doctor running the trial knows which of the two I am getting, hence we are "doubly blind"). The last part of the trial involves everyone getting the agent. I may not know if I will experience a positive result until then.

I am hoping for a good outcome, but if it doesn't work I remain optimistic that it is only a matter of time before something is discovered that will help. Until then I firmly maintain that my psoriasis is not who I am, and that it will not dictate how I live my life.

Taking the Psychological Blows

I still may be painting a confusing portrait of my experience. First, I tell you how miserable my psoriasis is and then I tell you that it is not that bad. I finished the last section by indicating that I refuse to let psoriasis run my life. This sounds quite bold and it is generally true. Now, I will confuse you with the part that is not "generally" true, with a couple of examples of how psoriasis has affected my life.

First, consider experiences at the swimming pool or beach. When stripped down into bathing trunks, one has no place to hide. Polite Canadians generally do not comment on the red mess they see, but it is silly to try convincing yourself that they do not see it. I have, over the years, often taken a rebellious approach to this problem. I tell myself that "this is not a contagious disease, it cannot hurt anyone, and others are just going to have to live with me sharing their water." However, the swimming pool scene is more disconcerting than the beach, especially when signs saying "No Open Sores in Pool" are posted. Does this include me? And, if it doesn't include me in reality, would it include me in the perception of the managers and other bathers? What would I do if challenged? This one is easy to answer because I know I would fight back. So, what to do? Is fighting for my rights worth the embarrassment to me, to the managers, to the bathers, to my nine-year-old son? Well, over the last couple of years my answer has been no. So, when my son asks, "Dad, will you swim with me?" I defer to supervising his solo swim.

Part of the problem with psoriasis, in my experience, is that Canadians are just too polite. People typically glance and then quickly look away, clearly embarrassed and uneasy. I often want to explain the condition to them, but seldom do. I do know firsthand that an explanation often provides a ready fix to whatever discomfort they and I are experiencing. This is another good reason to celebrate the innocence of children, who ask directly about my problem. As their parents try to pull them away in horror, I jump in and indicate that I am quite happy to explain. Children are generally satisfied with the explanation, and the situation is quickly diffused for the parent and me. Of course, I am not critical of this Canadian sensibility per se as I value manners highly. At the same time, a simple question would be so much more preferable. Other cultures are not as concerned about this particular brand of "manners," as much of my work in developing nations has demonstrated. In the countries I visit, adults quite readily ask me about my problem. A brief explanation sets things right immediately, though I often have to listen to an extended sales pitch for their homegrown remedies.

My recent divorce provided another significant challenge, one of which I am sure that many others with psoriasis are already well aware. How does one who is already feeling rejected and vulnerable find the spirit to risk rejection because of appearance? For me, the problem was not particularly pronounced so long as I dated only in the winter (when I would be clothed head to toe) and provided that I had no interest in being romantic. This, of course, is not realistic or even desirable. The process had to start by telling myself some things that I didn't really believe like "I have a lot to offer and she will be able to see beyond skin deep. If she can't do that, then I'm not interested in her anyway." I retained hope that someone might grow to find me attractive given enough contact, but how could someone get over that initial hump when physical appearance seems to trump character? I just could not convince myself that appearance would not matter.

Anyway, I forged ahead with this false bravado mixed with a great deal of apprehension. It is my good fortune to have met a special person who is able to see beyond the outward appearance. In her words, "it's only dry skin." Well, of course she is mostly right about this, but I know that her eye must catch more than a little bit of dry skin. I am grateful for her generosity of spirit and would like to think that I would behave in the same way had our roles been reversed. But would I? I know what the answer should be, but I worry that the answer that should be is not the answer that would be.

A More Professional Look
My interest in psoriasis shifted several years ago from the purely personal to the professional. I work as a university-based researcher and clinical psychologist, so the idea of how other people experienced their psoriasis intrigued me. I collaborated with Dr. Sandy Murray, Ms. Janet Lowe (both dermatology associates in Halifax), Dr. Cynthia Mathieson (Mount Saint Vincent University), and Dr. Karen Ruggiero (formerly of Harvard University) to answer this question with the help of about 100 people receiving light treatments for their psoriasis. As two of the resulting published studies are some of the most recent in the scientific literature, I thought that sharing some of the results here might be useful.

What Is Physical and What Is Psychological?
Our findings showed that people think in more than one way about the negative effects of psoriasis. Most people make a clear distinction between what bothers them psychologically (what we call psychosocial impact) and what bothers them physically (how much people can do on a daily basis). Although this may seem obvious, it seems important to note that two very different thought processes come into play when considering this disease. On the physical side, people reported different degrees of distress about how much pain, stinging, and itching they experienced. Psychosocial distress involved

other people noticing their psoriasis, disruptions to social life, and disruptions to daily routines. It was interesting that the amount of scaling on the skin was associated with psychological distress and not physical impact.

Gender Differences

It is generally accepted that physical appearance counts for more in the lives of women than in the lives of men. It is often assumed that this general truth extends to those with psoriasis, even though previous studies have failed to provide clear evidence of a more negative experience for women. Our survey provided some mixed findings on this point. Women did report that they faced more discrimination because of their psoriasis than did men, a conclusion with which the men in our study agreed. However, when asked more directly about how stigmatizing their experience with psoriasis has been (including feelings of self-worth), there was little to distinguish between men and women about how negatively the disease had affected their lives. One of the many potential implications of our findings is the need to exercise caution when applying stereotypes to the experiences of others. It may be that all of the participants recognized that women should be more affected than men, but the reality may be that men and women cope (or fail to cope) equally with the disease. The findings also suggested that for most people, psoriasis is hardly a "show stopper" in their lives. Human beings are quite resourceful, resilient, and able to cope with whatever life serves up.

Age Differences

Older people surveyed reported that their psoriasis had a greater general psychosocial impact on their lives than did younger participants. We found this somewhat surprising as we expected the opposite. On the other hand, younger participants had greater feelings of guilt about their psoriasis than did older respondents.

We thought the degree to which psoriasis bothers people might not vary just on the basis of age when surveyed, but also on the basis of age when first diagnosed. Children and especially teenagers face the challenge of developing a sense of identity. We can all remember how important appearance and "fitting in" was during our junior and senior high school years. We found those participants who were diagnosed at relatively earlier ages reported they were more sensitive and afraid of rejection than were those diagnosed later in life. It is important to remember that this finding did not relate to the *current* age of participants. It seems that those diagnosed earlier in life had greater trouble shaking off negative feelings about themselves as they grew older. This finding supports the fact that when facing psoriasis when you are young, the effects are lasting. Doctors and parents should be aware of the vulnerability of those coping with psoriasis when it strikes during the critical periods of identity formation and peer comparisons that occur during the teenage years.

Severity

We were somewhat surprised to find that the severity of psoriasis, measured by the standard instrument dermatologists use, was not strongly linked to how negatively psoriasis had impacted participants' lives. The exception was for a number of participants with very severe conditions who were more likely to reach out to support groups. This finding doesn't mean that severity is irrelevant. One must consider that the people surveyed were all living with a significant degree of severity as indicated by their receiving light treatments. The situation of these participants might be quite different from those who experience milder forms of the disease. Still, this finding suggests that how one feels about his or her psoriasis is a very subjective and individual experience, so there is no right or wrong way to feel about your condition. It is important that the negative effects of psoriasis be dealt with on an individual, not a "one size fits all," basis.

What You Can Do
Psoriasis is a chronic skin disease that disrupts daily life based on the necessity of ongoing medical treatment, the physical discomfort, and the pain that accompanies the condition. Even more important, at least for most of us, is the effect the disease has on our appearance and in how we present ourselves to the outside world.

It is important to remember that others' perception of our physical appearance may not be the same as the appearance that we think we project. Although it is silly to think that others do not notice our condition or that their judgment of us is never influenced by outward appearance, we can easily slip into patterns of hypersensitivity, where we overestimate how negatively others view us. If we present ourselves to others in ways that betray insecurity or unnecessary fear about prejudicial treatment, we risk damaging our social relationships much more than would be the case based only on our physical appearance.

Psychologists often emphasize the importance of "self-talk" in helping us cope with stressful or uncomfortable situations. In this light it is necessary that we keep reminding ourselves that psoriasis is a condition we live with, but it is not a defining characteristic of who we are as people. Of course, "self-talk" is cheap; it is one thing to tell ourselves that psoriasis is no big deal, but quite another to actually believe it. However, we will be more likely to believe it the more we tell ourselves that we are much more than a collection of blotchy red spots and scaling skin.

Earlier I mentioned the importance of feelings of control for psychological well-being. This need for control leaves many of us obsessed with finding a cure. This is probably not a useful strategy. With some chronic diseases, chronic pain being the most notable, the search for a cure actually worsens the condition. People with chronic pain often experience a significant degree of pain relief once they accept that the pain will remain a part of their lives. This is not to say that we shouldn't remain optimistic about an eventual cure because the current flurry of research activities investigating new treatments provides much reason for optimism. However, we are not there yet, and we would be wise to accept the old saying about accepting the things we cannot change.

However, accepting the reality of our condition is not the same as being passive. We can achieve a sense of control by actively pursuing the options that are available to us, and we will likely achieve an improvement in our symptoms. Obsessively seeking a cure is not helpful; active coping is.

There are many ways to cope, and I do not intend to exhaust them here. One thing we can do is seek support from others who share our experience through the many support groups that exist. Another way to actively cope is to pursue, in consultation with our doctors, the variety of new treatment opportunities that are now opening up. Considering a change in lifestyle may also be helpful. Although we no longer think that unhealthy living habits and psychological stress are the root causes of psoriasis, it seems likely that these factors can worsen our conditions. We can also do ourselves a favor by being active collaborators with our doctors, which moves us beyond the role of "patient" to the role of an active problem solver. One way to do this is to keep ourselves educated about the nature of our condition and of the emerging findings that provide us with the means by which to enhance the quality of our lives. In reading this book, you have already demonstrated your interest in education and in being an active coper. What else can you do to help yourself?

- *Get educated:* Learn as much as possible about psoriasis so you can better understand the disease and achieve realistic expectations.
- *Find a doctor who works for you:* Finding the right doctor and developing a good relationship is important to positive treatment results.
- *Communicate:* Communicating your feelings to your doctor, family, and peers will help improve your life and your relationships.
- *Give treatment a chance:* Certain medications take weeks to kick in. Be patient. Don't give up hope.
- Take time to relax and enjoy stress-free moments.
- Be positive!
- Seek a support group.
- See "Further Resources" (page 188).

Psoriasis Disability Index†
(† © A.Y. Finlay, 1993)

The Psoriasis Disability Index is intended for patients 16 years and older, and consists of fifteen simple, disease-specific questions. Each question is graded from 0 to 4, resulting in a maximum score of 45. The overall score suggests the impact that psoriasis has had on the patient during the last four weeks. This score is used to show changes in disability following treatment. The scoring of each question is based on a four-point scale:

Not at all = 0   A little = 1   A lot = 2   Very much = 3

When totaled, the score from each of the questions results in a maximum of 45 and a minimum of 0.

A low score reflects that psoriasis has had little effect; a high score reflects a significant impact and indicates that a visit to the doctor is advisable. There are many excellent support services and treatments available to treat this disease, and reason for hope in the future.

Each question relates to the last four weeks only.

Daily Activities

1. In the last four weeks, how much has your psoriasis interfered with you carrying out work around the house or garden?
   Not at all   A little   A lot   Very much

2. Over the last four weeks, how often have you worn different types or colors of clothes because of your psoriasis?
   Not at all   A little   A lot   Very much

3. Over the last four weeks, how much more have you had to change or wash your clothes?
   Not at all   A little   A lot   Very much

4. Over the last four weeks, how much of a problem has your psoriasis been at the hairdresser's?
   Not at all   A little   A lot   Very much

5. Over the last four weeks, how much has your psoriasis resulted in you having to take more baths than usual?
   Not at all   A little   A lot   Very much

If usually working, please answer questions 6a and 7a, then go to question 8. If you are not working, please answer questions 6b and 7b.

6. (a) How much has your psoriasis made you lose time from work over the last four weeks?
   (b) How much has your psoriasis stopped you from carrying out your normal daily activities over the last four weeks?
   Not at all   A little   A lot   Very much

7. (a) How much has your psoriasis prevented you from doing things at work or school over the last four weeks?
   (b) How much has your psoriasis altered the way in which you carry out your normal daily activities over the last four weeks?
   Not at all   A little   A lot   Very much

8. Has your career been affected by your psoriasis (e.g., promotion refusal, lost a job, asked to change a job)?
   Not at all   A little   A lot   Very much

Personal Relationships
9. Has your psoriasis resulted in sexual difficulties over the last four weeks?
   Not at all   A little   A lot   Very much

10. Has your psoriasis created problems with your partner or any of your close friends or relatives over the last four weeks?
    Not at all   A little   A lot   Very much

Leisure
11. Over the last four weeks, how much has your psoriasis stopped you from going out socially or to any function?
    Not at all   A little   A lot   Very much

12. Over the last four weeks, has your psoriasis made it difficult to do any sports?

   Not at all   A little   A lot   Very much

13. Have you been unable to use, been criticized for, or stopped from using communal bathing or changing facilities over the last four weeks?

   Not at all   A little   A lot   Very much

14. Over the last four weeks, has your psoriasis resulted in you smoking or drinking alcohol more than you would normally?

   Not at all   A little   A lot   Very much

Treatment

15. To what extent has your psoriasis or treatment made your home messy or untidy over the last four weeks?

   Not at all   A little   A lot   Very much

EIGHT

Introduction to Treatment Approaches

There are four main types of treatments for psoriasis, each of which will be explained and discussed in the following chapters:

- topical treatment
- phototherapy
- systemic therapy
- biologics

Some patients might use only one type of therapy, while others could use a combination.

The type(s) of therapy used depends on many factors; the treatments prescribed for each patient can be highly individualized—what works for some will not necessarily work for all. Sometimes finding the right treatment is a process of trial and error. Given the increasing options for psoriasis therapy, psoriasis experts wanted to establish a way for doctors to diagnose, categorize, and prescribe a treatment for psoriasis based on its type and severity. To expedite such a system, a group of psoriasis and psoriatic arthritis experts from the United States and Canada organized a psoriasis education therapy conference under the support of the American Academy of Dermatology and the National Psoriasis Foundation in November 2002 in Louisville, Kentucky. There, a consensus statement and guidelines of care for the management of psoriasis were developed.

Here is a list of factors that doctors and patients can take into account before starting a specific treatment. Disease-related factors that could influence the effectiveness of a particular therapy include:

- type of psoriasis (e.g., chronic plaque-type versus pustular psoriasis)
- extent of disease (e.g., localized versus widespread)
- area affected (e.g., hands or feet can be disabled and require more aggressive therapy)
- location (e.g., more sensitive areas—groin or armpits—may require different treatments)

Patient-related factors also control which therapy will work best. These include:

- lifestyle
- occupation
- geographic location (if at a distance from treatment centers, it could be difficult for the patient to receive certain therapies, such as phototherapy)
- other health problems that require medication (certain psoriasis medications might interact with other medications)

In the past, dermatologists have classified patients according to the severity of their disease based on the amount or extent of psoriasis. Classifications for psoriasis included mild, moderate, or severe, depending on how much of the patient's body surface area was affected.

- If less than 10 percent of the body surface area was involved, the patient was classified as having mild to moderate disease.
- If more than 10 percent of the body surface area was involved, the patient was classified as having moderate to severe disease.
- If more than 30 percent of body surface area was affected, a patient was deemed to have severe psoriasis.

This method is now falling out of favor for several reasons.

Basing the severity of disease on the extent of involvement alone fails to recognize other important factors that can impact the severity of disease. For example, factors such as the location of lesions (face, hands, or feet), resistance to prior therapies, and the impact on social and emotional well-being of affected people are very important, as is the impact on their quality of life. Some of the key aspects that determine quality of life include:

- physical factors, such as the severity of itching, irritation, pain, insomnia, or inability to use the hands or feet
- psychological factors, such as the degree of a patient's self-consciousness, embarrassment, frustration, anger, helplessness, depression, stigmatization, and anticipation of rejection
- social impact, such as the fear of going to social functions, shaking hands, and wearing certain types of clothing to hide lesions
- sexual impact, including feelings of physical unattractiveness leading to less sexual activity
- occupational impact, such as being eliminated from certain jobs, lost days of work due to psoriasis, and loss of productivity due to time-consuming treatment schedules

Drug Interactions

For those taking oral or injectable therapies, it is important to educate yourself about drug interactions, especially those that could interact with your treatment regime. For example, certain drugs can reduce the effectiveness of the therapy or increase the chance of side effects. Please see specific treatments in the following chapters for more specific exact drug interactions.

Depending on the above considerations, your doctor will discuss all possible treatments with you. You will be monitored while on the therapy; however, if you feel the treatment is ineffective, irritating, or very inconvenient, you should discuss alternatives with your doctor.

Goals of Therapy

Define the goal of therapy with your doctor so that together you can determine if it is realistic and matches the type of therapy you are currently receiving. Although complete clearing of psoriasis is achievable with some new therapies, it should be understood that in many cases complete clearance might not be possible. What is possible is significant improvement by clearing a large portion of the disease. However, it is important to remember that because psoriasis is not currently curable, the disease usually does come back after clearance or near clearance is obtained.

The time it takes for psoriasis to clear depends on a number of factors, which range from the type(s) of therapy being used to the type and degree of psoriasis that presents. In addition, maintenance therapy (the therapy that continues after initial improvement) might be required. Depending on the patient and the doctor, the therapy used can range from topicals to phototherapy to systemics to biologics.

NINE

Topical Therapies

Topical treatments (applied directly to the skin) are the first medications most often prescribed by doctors for patients with psoriasis. These treatments are used alone for mild disease, or in combination with phototherapy or systemic therapy for moderate to severe disease. Topical medications are typically used when psoriasis involves only a few areas or is not creating discomfort for the patient. In patients with mild disease, such therapies can be quite effective in controlling the signs and symptoms of psoriasis. These therapies are generally not effective when used alone in patients with more severe disease; for these patients, topicals can be used in addition to phototherapy or systemic therapy. Also, topicals can be used after psoriasis clears or nearly clears to maintain the improvement of the disease while off phototherapy or systemic therapy.

Components/Ingredients of Topicals

A *vehicle* or *base* is the substance into which the active medication is inserted so that it can be transported to the outer layer of skin or through the skin's surface to the site of inflammation. In topical therapies different bases or vehicles are used, including:

- creams
- ointments
- lotions

- gels
- aerosols

Creams often appear white, and dissolve well into the skin. Ointments tend to be almost clear and greasy, like petroleum jelly. Ointments also tend to be more lubricating and are more potent than creams containing the same concentration of active medication. Lotions are liquid-like preparations, gels are jelly-like material, and aerosols can be applied topically as a fine mist.

How Much Are You Supposed to Use?

A practical measure of the amount of topical medication to use on a body area was developed in 1991 by Dr. Long and Dr. Finlay at the University of Wales College of Medicine, Cardiff. They came up with the fingertip unit (FTU) to enable doctors and patients to communicate better about the amount of medication to apply. A fingertip unit is the amount of cream squeezed out of a tube that covers the skin from the tip of the index finger to the first crease in the finger's skin. It is possible to relate a fingertip unit to a body site to accurately determine how much topical treatment to use. For example, in adults, 1 FTU would be required for the hand only; 2 FTUs for one foot; 3 FTUs for one arm; 6 FTUs for one leg, and 7 FTUs for the front or back of the trunk.

Moisturizers

Moisturizers are an important tool in treating and controlling mild psoriasis, at least partially. However, they are seldom able to control and treat psoriasis when used alone, particularly in more severe psoriasis. They can help relieve mild itching and dry skin, and can reduce scaling or flaking of the skin. Moisturizers or emollients provide a surface barrier on the skin that slows its dehydration and keeps it moist. In general, moisturizers are applied twice daily, but they can be used more frequently, particularly if dry, flaking skin is noted. There are many moisturizers available over the counter at a pharmacy. Moisturizers, such as petroleum jelly and glycerin, are useful for moisturizing the skin. If you're not sure what to buy, ask your doctor or the pharmacist.

Topical Steroids

Topical steroids are anti-inflammatory medications that reduce skin inflammation in psoriasis. Topical steroid creams can help control the itch of psoriasis and decrease the thickness of the outer layer of the skin. Corticosteroids are the most commonly prescribed topical therapy for the management of psoriasis and are available in several forms, including ointments, creams, lotions, aerosols, or tapes (in the United States). An advantage of topical steroids is that they work relatively quickly and the cost is quite reasonable.

Steroid Potencies

Topical steroids range from low to high or ultra-high potency. Ointments are usually more potent than creams that contain the same concentration and type of steroid.

In general, doctors may start psoriasis patients using low to mid-potency steroids. The strength and base (i.e., ointment or cream) of the steroid used may vary according to the site and the type of psoriasis lesions. For example, thick plaques of psoriasis on the elbows and knees may require higher potencies in an ointment form in order to penetrate the thick skin in these locations. Salicylic acid may be combined with the topical steroid as it reduces the scaling and can help increase steroid penetration. On the other hand, doctors generally like to use low-potency steroids in very sensitive areas where the skin is thin, such as in the genital region, the face (e.g., eyelids), and folds (crease between the buttocks, under the arms and breasts).

Most topical steroids are available by prescription only. Only milder topical steroids (e.g., hydrocortisone 0.5 percent) are available from the pharmacist without a prescription. Examples of some of the different types of corticosteroids that are available as creams, ointments, gels, foams, lotions, and solutions are listed below according to their potencies.

Topical Corticosteroids Classified According to Potency

Class	Potency	Examples
Class 1	Superpotent (ultra-high)	Clobetasol 17-propionate (Dermovate®) 0.05% (cream/ointment)
		Betamethasone dipropionate (Diprosone®) 0.05% (ointment)
		Halobetasol propionate (Ultravate®) 0.05% (cream/ointment)
Class 2	Potent (high to ultra-high)	Betamethasone dipropionate 0.05% (cream)
		Mometasone furoate (Elocom®) 0.1% (ointment)
		Fluocinonide (Lyderm®; Tiamol®; Lidex®;) 0.05% (cream/ointment)
Class 3	Potent (high)	Betamethasone dipropionate 0.05% (cream)
Class 4	Mid-strength (medium to high)	Betamethasone valerate (Betaderm®; Prevex B®) 0.1% (ointment)
		Mometasone furoate 0.1% (cream)
Class 5	Mid-strength (medium)	Betamethasone valerate 0.1% (cream)
		Fluocinolone acetonide (Synalar®) 0.025% (cream)
		Betamethasone valerate 0.05% (cream)
Class 6	Mild (low to medium)	Desonide (Desocort®) 0.05% (cream)
Class 7	Mild (low)	Hydrocortisone (Cortoderm®; Emo-Cort®; Hycort®; Hydrosone®; Prevex HC®) 0.5% and 1% (cream/ointment)

What Are the Possible Complications of Topical Steroids?

Steroids have been used extensively for long periods and are very safe when used appropriately. However, topical steroids can have certain side effects when they are either highly potent or used over long periods, and when used in more sensitive areas where the skin is thin.

Tips for Topical Steroid Therapy

- If you have very thick, scaly lesions, it might be necessary to apply salicylic acid (either in combination with a topical steroid, or in a topical cream or ointment as prescribed by your doctor) to reduce the scales and enable the active medication to penetrate the skin better.
- If you are applying it on very thin skin (such as the genitals or face), check with a doctor or pharmacist that the potency of the steroid you are using is right for you.
- Avoid applying stronger steroids to the face or skin folds unless instructed by a doctor. Also, make sure you know how long your doctor wants you to use them (usually only a few weeks), especially when applied to these sensitive areas.

The most common side effects reported with prolonged use of potent corticosteroids are stretch marks (striae) and thinning of the skin (atrophy). Both of these side effects occur with prolonged use of treatment (after at least one month of continual use), and tend to occur in areas where the skin is more sensitive or thin, especially the armpits and groin. Thinning of the skin is usually reversible if caught early and treatment is stopped. Stretch marks can also occur and are usually irreversible. Other side effects include:

- increased darkening of the skin (hyperpigmentation)
- increased lightening of the skin (hypopigmentation)
- acne (perioral acne)
- acne-like eruptions (rosacea)
- contact or irritant dermatitis
- easy bruising (purpura)
- inflammation of the hair follicle (folliculitis)
- increased blood vessel formation
- infection
- rebound of psoriasis (on stopping the treatment, usually abruptly)
- loss of response (tachyphylaxis)

Possible but rare side effects include:
- glaucoma (increased pressure in the eye)
- Cushing's syndrome (a hormonal disorder caused by prolonged exposure of the body's tissues to high levels of the hormone cortisol)
- decreased growth in children (very rare)

Never abruptly discontinue the use of potent topical steroids unless advised by your doctor or if you are having a reaction to the medication, or you might experience a rebound or flare-up of psoriasis or a temporary worsening of the lesions.

Some people might be unable to use topical steroids, particularly if they have any known allergy to corticosteroids or any component in it and/or any bacterial, fungal, or viral infections at the site of application.

In addition, topical steroids can lose their effect over time. This is termed "tachyphylaxis," meaning the body has developed a tolerance to the beneficial effects of the medication.

Coal Tar

Different types of coal tar are used to treat psoriasis-affected skin (shale, wood, coal, and distilled coal tar). Crude coal tar is one of the oldest psoriasis treatment options available. Many patients dislike using tar because it may be messy, smelly, and irritating. However, coal tar can provide significant benefit for patients.

Topical coal tar is available as a gel, cream, ointment, liquid, bath solution, or shampoo. Coal tar can stain white hair, clothing, towels, and bedding; therefore, if you apply it before going to bed, use old pajamas and bedding. Coal tar can make the skin more sensitive to sunlight (photosensitizer), so be careful when exposing your skin to sunlight the day of coal tar application and carefully follow your doctor's instructions.

Psoriasis treatment centers may prescribe the Goeckerman regimen (see Chapter 9), whereby coal tar is applied before exposure to ultraviolet-B light to enable the ultraviolet rays to have a greater therapeutic effect on the skin. Coal tar is also effective when combined with topical corticosteroids.

Anthralin

Anthralin (Psoriatec®) has been widely used in the past as an effective treatment for psoriasis, but is now prescribed less frequently because, like tar, it is messy and stains clothing. Anthralin is able to stop psoriatic skin cell turnover, has an anti-inflammatory effect, and is most effective on chronic plaque-type psoriasis.

Anthralin is available in different concentrations, and therapy usually starts at a low potency with a gradual increase in the strength until the desired effect is obtained. Psoriasis treatment centers may use the Ingram regimen (see Chapter 9), which involves applying anthralin prior to exposing the skin to ultraviolet-B light. The Ingram regimen is generally used to treat moderate to severe psoriasis.

Another method of treating psoriasis with anthralin involves short contact anthralin therapy (SCAT) with higher potencies of anthralin applied to the skin, kept on for a short period of time, and then washed off. Application time is generally increased with subsequent applications until the psoriasis lesions have improved.

Unfortunately, anthralin is very messy and can discolor the skin, hair, and clothes. Newer preparations that stain less are now available. Anthralin can also be irritating to the skin. After application, it is advisable to wash the hands carefully. It is also important that patients do not expose anthralin to sensitive body areas and other untreated areas. If anthralin gets in the eyes, irritation can occur.

Vitamin D Analogue: Calcipotriol

Calcipotriol (Dovonex®, Daivonex®) is a derivative of vitamin D that became available in Canada in 1991 and was subsequently approved for U.S. distribution. Vitamin D can slow the rate at which psoriatic skin cells multiply. Calcipotriol also has anti-inflammatory properties. This topical treatment can be found in ointment, cream, or solution form. Calcipotriol comes in one strength (0.005 percent) and is available in 60 and 120 gram tubes (cream and ointment) and 30 milliliter and 60 milliliter scalp solutions. It is typically applied once or twice daily to the affected area, and improvements are usually seen within four to eight weeks.

Its major advantage over topical steroids is that it is a nonsteroidal therapy and therefore lacks many of the possible local side effects seen with steroids, such as skin thinning.

Although calcipotriol is well tolerated, it does have some drawbacks: It is slow to take effect and may cause irritation after application, particularly on the face and in skin folds. Another rare side effect is an increase in the levels of calcium in the bloodstream. The risk of increased calcium levels (hypercalcemia) is not seen if the maximum dose of 100 grams of calcipotriol per week is not exceeded in adults.

Calcipotriol might need to be used in combination with another topical therapy, phototherapy, or systemic medications in order to improve effectiveness. In 2001, a combination of calcipotriol and betamethasone dipropionate in the treatment of chronic plaque-type psoriasis was investigated and proved very effective. Because this new combination treatment includes a high-potency topical steroid, it is generally used for shorter periods, usually once a day for one month. After that time, another topical therapy can be substituted. Recently, a scalp gel containing calcipotriol and betamethasone dipropionate (Xamiol) has been successfully used in patients with scalp psoriasis.

It is important to note that calcipotriol is inactivated by salicylic acid, and lesions should not be pretreated with such keratolytics.

Calcineurin Inhibitors (Nonsteroidal Therapies)

Calcineurin inhibitors (also known as topical immunomodulators or TIMs) are a new class of therapy that has been recently approved in the United States and Canada for the treatment of atopic dermatitis/eczema. Their use in treatment of psoriasis is being investigated. They work by inhibiting a key step in the activation of the T-lymphocyte, a cell in the immune system that is important in causing the skin changes of psoriasis and atopic dermatitis. There are two types of calcineurin inhibitors:

- tacrolimus (Protopic®) (0.1 percent and 0.03 percent ointment)
- pimecrolimus (Elidel®) (1 percent cream)

In the treatment of psoriasis, calcineurin inhibitors have had variable success. Initial clinical research failed to prove any benefit of topical tacrolimus or pimecrolimus in the treatment of psoriasis when applied to thick, scaly areas. There is evidence, however, that both these agents are effective when used for psoriasis on sites such as the face, groin, or armpits. These areas are particularly vulnerable to thinning of the skin when treated with topical steroids, which makes these new agents valuable additions as thinning of the skin has not been reported with either tacrolimus or pimecrolimus.

Since calcineurin inhibitors are nonsteroidal, they lack many of the side effects that can occur with topical steroids. The major side effect seen with tacrolimus or pimecrolimus is temporary burning on the skin. This tends to last for only a few minutes after application and generally resolves on its own within a week to ten days of therapy. Unfortunately, these agents are significantly more expensive than topical steroids.

Topical tacrolimus (Protopic®) is currently available in ointment form as a 0.03–0.1 percent concentration (10 gram, 30 gram, 60 gram, and 100 gram tubes). Topical pimecrolimus (Elidel®) is available in a 1 percent concentration cream (30 gram, 60 gram, and 100 gram tubes) only as a prescription.

Currently, there is ongoing clinical research to develop new bases such as creams, ointments, or gels. Pimecrolimus in pill form is currently being tested for use in chronic plaque-type psoriasis, and the initial clinical results have been very encouraging.

Tazarotene (Tazorac®)

Tazarotene is a topical vitamin A derivative available in a gel or cream. Tazarotene is effective predominantly in reducing scaling and thickness of plaques, but is less successful in reducing redness. When prescribed alone, the use of tazarotene is limited because many patients develop significant irritation at the site of application. Irritation can be reduced if tazarotene is used in combination with other topical steroids.

Tazarotene increases the skin's photosensitivity and has been successfully combined with both ultraviolet-B and narrow-band ultraviolet-B therapy to provide more effective and rapid clearing of psoriasis versus either treatment alone. Tazarotene should not be used during pregnancy.

TEN

Light Therapy

Natural sunlight is known to have a beneficial effect on patients with psoriasis. In rare instances, psoriasis patients might find that sunlight actually worsens their condition. Natural sunlight is composed of three types of radiation: ultraviolet (UV) radiation, the visible light spectrum, and infrared radiation. Visible light waves are the only light waves we can see, and we see them as colors of the rainbow. Infrared light cannot be seen. Longer infrared light waves can be felt as heat similar to that of the sun, fire, or a radiator. Short or near infrared light waves cannot be felt. Near infrared, for example, is used by a TV's remote control. Each category in the light spectrum comprises different components that have their own unique wavelength. The shorter the wavelength, the less energy the light source carries. Just as we measure distance with meters, we measure light waves using a wavelength measurement called nanometers. A wavelength is a measure of 1 nanometer. You would need 1 million nanometers just to make 1 millimeter.

UV light waves found in sunlight are the source of the beneficial effect on psoriasis. There are three types of ultraviolet rays in sunlight: UVC (110–290 nanometers), UVB (290–320 nanometers), and UVA (320–400 nanometers). UVC rays are blocked by the ozone layer and do not reach Earth's surface. UV therapy involves the use of UVA and/or UVB.

UVB rays are highly effective in treating psoriasis. UVB rays are known as sunburn (B = burning) rays because they represent the portion of sunlight that causes sunburns, and they are mainly responsible for changing skin color, such as when we tan (UVA can also play a role). UVB rays can improve psoriasis on their own or in combination with other treatments. UVA therapy is effective in treating psoriasis when combined with psoralen, but is not very effective when used alone.

Before you undertake a treatment program with phototherapy, it is important to understand how your skin will react to the light. Also, you must let your doctor know if you have any other health problems and what other medications you are on. Some health problems may prohibit you from receiving phototherapy (contraindications). Your doctor could decide that you should not be treated with phototherapy for one of the following reasons:

- You have another disease that causes your skin to be very sensitive to UV light (e.g., systemic lupus erythematosus, polymorphic light eruption).
- The medication(s) you take for your other medical conditions make your skin more sensitive to UV.
- You have a past history of melanoma (the most serious form of skin cancer of the pigment-producing cells in the skin, called melanocytes).

Your doctor could also decide to avoid phototherapy if you have a history of another type of skin cancer (such as squamous cell carcinoma or basal cell carcinoma); those with such a history are at a greater risk for developing new skin cancers when exposing themselves to the sun or artificial light sources, such as those used in phototherapy.

Phototherapy can increase the risk of skin cancer, particularly if used over long periods. If you are having regular phototherapy treatment for your psoriasis, you should also plan for regular skin examinations to be sure no such skin cancers have developed. In addition, if at any time you recognize any non-healing areas on your skin or new growths of concern, arrange to see your doctor. Excess UVL, especially PUVA, will accelerate the appearance of photo-aging of the skin.

Studies have shown that psoralen plus ultraviolet-A (PUVA) light treatment has been linked to the most serious form of skin cancer, cutaneous melanoma. However, this is rare and generally happens only when PUVA treatment is given over a prolonged period.

Prior to beginning treatment with UV light, your doctor will start therapy based on your skin type. Dr. Thomas Fitzpatrick defined skin type based on the skin's response to sunlight exposure. This method groups skin types from I to VI based on whether the skin burns or tans in response to sunlight exposure. This guideline is one method used to determine the starting dosage of ultraviolet therapy.

Skin Types and Their Effects When Exposed to Sunlight

Skin Type	Sunburns	Tans	Sun Sensitivity
I	Always	Never	Extreme
II	Easily	Sometimes	Very
III	Sometimes	Slowly	Moderate
IV	Minimally	Always	Slight
V	Seldom	Darkens	Barely
VI	Never	Darkens	Insensitive

A second method your doctor may use to determine your starting dose of ultraviolet radiation is through skin testing. This involves exposing small areas of skin sequentially to different intensities of ultraviolet-B radiation to see the response of your skin.

Ultraviolet-B Light Therapy

Ultraviolet-B rays are highly effective in treating psoriasis. Phototherapy with ultraviolet-B alone or in combination with other agents, such as coal tar or anthralin (Psoriatec®), can improve psoriasis. Ultraviolet-B can be given as:

- Ultraviolet-B (290–320 nanometers)—also known as broad-band UVB
- Narrow-band UVB (311 nanometers)
- Goeckerman regimen (UVB plus coal tar)
- Ingram regimen (UVB plus anthralin)
- UVB plus systemic agent
- UVB plus another topical agent (calcipotriol [Dovonex®, Daivonex®], tazarotene [Tazorex®], topical steroid)

The starting dose for each patient depends on his or her skin type, and typically ultraviolet-B treatments start with only a few seconds of exposure to light. Over time the exposure time is gradually increased until the skin is clear. You could require treatment anywhere from three to five times a week, and as your skin begins to clear, your doctor might stop light treatments or start you on a regular schedule to maintain your improvement. This can include coming in once every week, two weeks, or monthly. During your active treatment period, you will be examined on a regular basis by the treatment staff at the phototherapy unit. If you burn during treatment, immediately notify your dermatologist or the treatment staff.

Precautions to Take While Undergoing Ultraviolet-B Therapy

- Do not attend tanning beds while receiving light treatment.
- Cover up when outdoors or use a sunscreen (SPF 15+), especially on the days you receive light treatment and for the duration of the treatment.

- Use sunscreen during treatment on sensitive areas, such as nipples and lips.
- Men should shield their genital area when getting light treatments.

Combining Ultraviolet-B with Topical Agents

Goeckerman Regimen

Developed in 1925 by Dr. Goeckerman, the regimen named after him is a combination therapy of tar and UVB radiation. Tar can be highly effective in the treatment of psoriasis when combined with ultraviolet-B because tar makes the skin more sensitive (photosensitizes) to ultraviolet light. Together, tar and UVB can help slow the high turnover of skin cells, and reduce inflammation and itching.

While there have been many modifications to the Goeckerman regimen, this procedure in general calls for the application of distilled coal tar before exposure to ultraviolet light, followed by a bath after exposure to remove any excess tar:

- Distilled coal tar is applied by topical application, or by taking a tar bath, before exposure to UVB radiation.
- Have exposure to UVB phototherapy according to the dose determined by the treatment staff.
- Take a plain soap-and-water bath to remove excess tar. Do not rub vigorously to remove it.
- If this process is to be repeated the next day, you might be asked to apply tar and a stockinette suit or sauna suit, which is left on until the next day, before leaving the treatment center.

The Goeckerman regimen is one of the most effective methods of inducing a temporary clearance of psoriasis; however, it has several disadvantages: The tar is messy and causes staining and discoloration of the skin, and the regimen is inconvenient.

Ingram Regimen

Dr. Ingram pioneered the use of anthralin with UVB. Anthralin and ultraviolet-B work together to help remove psoriasis plaques and stop the rapid turnover of skin cells, which, in part, causes the raised areas of skin in psoriasis. The regimen varies in each center, but the general principles involve the application of a 0.1–2 percent anthralin cream before exposure to ultraviolet radiation.

Anthralin is applied and covered by a stockinette or sauna suit the day before UVB treatment. At the treatment center, do the following:

- Remove anthralin paste by dabbing all areas with mineral oil and wiping off.
- Bathe in a tar bath (cup of coal tar solution in bath water) for ten minutes using soap.
- Dry off.
- Have exposure to UVB phototherapy.

The anthralin paste is then reapplied and covered with a stockinette or sauna suit.

Anthralin can stain clothes and bed linens permanently, so patients are advised to wear old clothing and use old linen. Also, the eyes and normal skin are extremely sensitive to anthralin and can quickly become irritated. Always wash your hands carefully after contact with anthralin.

Calcipotriol Plus UVB

In combination with ultraviolet-B, calcipotriol has been found to be highly effective in controlling psoriasis. The combination of calcipotriol with twice weekly UVB phototherapy may reduce the amount of ultraviolet-B required without using any other combinations. Unlike tar, calcipotriol is applied after ultraviolet-B exposure.

Tazarotene
Tazarotene has also been used with UVB; again the combination may work better than the sole use of UVB.

Combining Ultraviolet-B with Systemic Agents
Ultraviolet-B can also be combined with systemic agents, including methotrexate (Rheumatrex®), cyclosporine (Sandimmune®), and retinoids. Depending on the individual, any of these combinations could increase the effectiveness of therapy (see Chapter 11).

Home Ultraviolet-B Therapy
Ultraviolet therapy can be done at home using equipment that can be purchased through several distributors in the United States. If you are thinking about starting a program of ultraviolet-B therapy at home, first meet with your dermatologist to see if this is an appropriate option for you. If you are a suitable candidate for this therapy, your dermatologist will provide you with a prescription for the light panels.

Home therapy must be carefully monitored so that excessive exposure to ultraviolet light (which can increase your risk of skin cancer) is avoided, and to ensure the proper dosage is chosen and used to avoid burning.

Home therapy is rare in North America because, understandably, many dermatologists are reluctant to prescribe a treatment that is difficult to monitor and that has potential risks. Generally, only those who live far from treatment centers use home phototherapy. In addition, home phototherapy units are quite expensive.

Narrow-Band Ultraviolet-B Therapy

Also known as selective UVB phototherapy, narrow-band ultraviolet-B (NB-UVB) light therapy is a newer phototherapy method that can offer safer and more effective results in the treatment of psoriasis. Ultraviolet-B ranges from 290–320 nanometers in wavelength. Special narrow-band UVB lamps emit a very narrow band of high intensity light at 311–312 nanometer wavelengths.

The major advantage of this therapy is that it eliminates much of the high-energy, shorter ultraviolet-B wavelengths that have been attributed to burning, premature aging, and increased risk of skin cancers. Initial research has found that narrow-band ultraviolet-B is more effective and can keep the psoriasis clear for longer, even after the therapy is discontinued. Recent studies show that in some patients, narrow-band ultraviolet-B provides faster clearance with fewer treatments. For most, approximately 30–35 treatments could be required to obtain clearance; however, for some, it could be fewer.

Narrow-band ultraviolet-B can also be used in combination with topical treatments such as corticosteroids, calcipotriol, anthralin, tar, and tazarotene gel to improve psoriasis.

Psoralen Plus Ultraviolet-A Light Therapy

When used alone, ultraviolet-A is only minimally effective in treating psoriasis. However, when combined with topical application or ingestion of psoralen, ultraviolet-A can have a significantly greater effect in clearing psoriasis. Psoralen plus ultraviolet-A (PUVA) involves administering psoralen prior to exposing skin to ultraviolet-A light. Psoralen makes the skin more sensitive to the effect of ultraviolet light, and as a result improves the effect of ultraviolet-A in the treatment of psoriasis.

Dr. Parish, Dr. Fitzpatrick, and colleagues at Harvard Medical School first reported the use of PUVA in 1974. In their initial clinical experiment, a patient ingested psoralen, then half the body was covered and the patient received ultraviolet-A on the opposite side. The patient showed clearance of psoriasis on the side that received the combination, but no improvement on the side that was protected from UVA. This indicated that the combination of psoralen and ultraviolet-A was essential for obtaining the beneficial effect.

After taking psoralen, you need to wear protective sunglasses for twenty-four hours because there is a possible risk of developing cataracts (abnormalities in the lens of the eye, causing blurry vision or decreased vision). To date, an increase of cataracts has not been reported in PUVA patients treated with careful eye protection.

Certain patients should not have PUVA therapy, such as those with medical conditions that make them more sensitive to the sun (e.g., systemic lupus erythematosus). Also, if you are unable to stand for long periods of time, are pregnant, or are unable to comply with treatment, you should not use PUVA.

Reasons a Psoriasis Patient Should Not Receive PUVA Therapy
- history of skin cancer, particularly malignant melanoma
- systemic lupus erythematosus
- history of reaction to psoralen
- pregnant or nursing
- prior treatment with X-rays
- use of medication that makes the patient more sensitive to ultraviolet light (check with your doctor)

Sometimes PUVA is the only treatment that works for an individual; however, because it has potential short-term and long-term side effects, it is important to follow your doctor's

guidelines:
- Your doctor will record the amount of PUVA you receive and try to keep it under a certain amount.
- Eyes, nipples, lips, and genitals must be protected during PUVA treatments.

Before your doctor prescribes PUVA therapy, the following steps will generally occur:
1. evaluation by your doctor to determine if PUVA therapy would be beneficial
2. assessment of any reasons you should not have PUVA (contraindications)
3. full skin examination
4. eye examination, which will be repeated yearly
5. recording of any other medications you are taking to make sure no drugs that increase your sensitivity to the sun are being used (photosensitizing medications)

Should your doctor decide that PUVA is right for you, she or he will review PUVA with you and might ask you to sign a consent form (outlining the risks and benefits of treatment) before administering treatment. The PUVA treatment protocol can differ from center to center. The two most common schedules are to administer the therapy two or three times weekly. Your dermatologist will decide how the psoralen is administered (by mouth, bath, or applying psoralen directly to a given area).

If the disease is localized, such as on the hands or feet, a bath or topical PUVA is often used. Instead of taking a pill, patients either soak in a psoralen bath for 10–20 minutes or apply a psoralen cream 2 hours prior to ultraviolet-A exposure.

Both these methods have the advantage of avoiding some of the side effects of oral psoralen (e.g., nausea). These side effects are fewer because the medication is not taken orally and therefore does not enter the bloodstream.

Medication	Administered	After UVA Treatment	Common Side Effects
Oral PUVA 8-methoxypsoralen	1 to 2 hours before light treatment	Wear clothing/sunscreen to protect from sun. Wear protective eyewear for the next 24 hours	Nausea, dry skin, tanning, skin aging
Topical PUVA 8-methoxypsoralen cream	2 hours before light treatment	Wash off medication; put on sunscreen	Dry skin, tanning on UVA-exposed areas, increased sensitivity to sunlight after treatment
Bath PUVA 8-methoxypsoralen (0.5–1.0 mg/L)	Soak in bath for 10 minutes before light treatment	Shower/bathe to wash off medication; put on sunscreen	Dry skin, tanning

In general, the following steps will occur in orally administered PUVA therapy:

1. An oral dose of psoralen is given 2 hours prior to exposure to UV light.
2. Genitalia must be covered.
3. The eyes must be completed shielded by protective goggles.
4. UVA exposure occurs in a light machine (the dosage is based on your skin type).
5. UV protective sunglasses must be worn after treatment, especially outdoors. Exposure to sunlight should be minimal.
6. UVA may be increased (increased time in the light machine with subsequent sessions).
7. PUVA is given two or three times weekly until the desired effect is obtained.
8. If your skin reddens, the treatment could be canceled, or if redness is localized, the area can be shielded with clothing or zinc oxide.
9. Once clear, you may be placed on a maintenance schedule that requires you to return on a less frequent but regular basis.

10. On nontreatment days, exposure to sunlight should be minimized; outdoor use of sunglasses is also encouraged.

PUVA therapy generally shows improvement in the skin lesions within six to ten treatments. Clearance can often be obtained after twenty to thirty treatments, providing that treatments are not missed and instructions are followed.

Combination Therapy with PUVA

PUVA may be combined with another topical or oral treatment to increase the improvement in psoriasis at the same or lower dose of UVA radiation.

Acitretin (Retinoid) Plus PUVA (RePUVA)

Acitretin (Soriatane®) is an oral vitamin A analogue, or retinoid (see Chapter 10) that is given in combination with PUVA. Your doctor will usually start you on acitretin ten to fourteen days before beginning PUVA therapy. This therapy can be of particular use to those who have:

• failed PUVA therapy alone
• certain types of psoriasis (erythrodermic or generalized pustular)
• darker complexions

Pregnant women or women planning a pregnancy should not receive acitretin.

Methotrexate Plus PUVA

Methotrexate can also be used in combination with PUVA, a therapy that has been successful in certain patients with severe psoriasis and psoriatic arthritis. The patient can begin methotrexate two to three weeks before PUVA therapy. Take methotrexate exactly as directed by your doctor. Methotrexate is reviewed in detail in Chapter 11.

Balneotherapy (Climatotherapy)

The use of highly concentrated saltwater (greater than 20 percent) with ultraviolet light is known as balneotherapy. Balneotherapy first emerged as a treatment for various skin disorders in Europe in the 1800s.

The Dead Sea in Israel is one place balneotherapy is practiced. The Dead Sea has been known to be of therapeutic benefit for psoriasis patients. There are several scientific reasons for this: The Dead Sea lies 1,312 feet (400 meters) below sea level and UVB rays are largely filtered out, leaving a higher concentration of UVA rays, thereby allowing patients to expose their skin for long periods without burning. Also, the Dead Sea contains both salt (in concentrations ten times higher than ocean water) and a number of other minerals, such as magnesium, calcium, potassium, and bromine. These minerals seem to enhance the beneficial effects of the UVA.

Patients typically go to the Dead Sea, bathe in the water, and expose themselves to the sunlight for several weeks. Many return every year for relief of their psoriasis.

ELEVEN

Systemic Therapies

Systemic drugs are medications that are given either orally (pills) or as injections just below the skin (subcutaneous) or into the muscle (intramuscular). Since these medications enter the body's circulatory system directly, they are called systemic agents, and are usually reserved for patients with moderate to severe psoriasis, or for those with psoriatic arthritis. In addition, these medications are also used in combination with other therapies, including topicals and phototherapies, especially when a patient does not respond to a single type of treatment.

Currently, the most commonly used systemic agents for the treatment of psoriasis are methotrexate (Rheumatrex®), cyclosporine (Sandimmune®), and retinoids. These medications can provide significant benefit in clearing psoriasis, but they can have side effects. These side effects might occur either at the outset or shortly after starting the medication (acute side effects) or after prolonged use (long-term, chronic side effects). While on these medications, it is important to be closely monitored by your doctor. When taking any systemic agent, it is vital that the drug is taken as directed by your doctor.

Methotrexate (MTX)
Methotrexate is a medication initially developed and approved to treat different types of cancer (chemotherapy). Methotrex-

ate is also used to treat moderate to severe psoriasis and disabling psoriatic arthritis.

How Does Methotrexate Work?

Methotrexate is effective in erythrodermic, pustular, and severe plaque-type psoriasis, as well as psoriatic arthritis. Methotrexate is effective because it works in two major ways:

1. It reduces the rapid turnover of the skin cells, an important process in producing the thick, scaling lesions of psoriasis.
2. It has an anti-inflammatory effect on white blood cells (activated T-cells), which are important in the development of psoriasis lesions (and suppression of the immune system).

Patients Who May Benefit from Methotrexate

- those with erythrodermic psoriasis (entire body is covered by red scaling lesions)
- those with pustular psoriasis (generalized or localized such as palmoplantar pustulosis)
- those with plaque-type psoriasis (involving the hands, feet, face) or extensive body areas
- those with psoriatic arthritis
- those who fail to respond to topical therapies, phototherapy, or other systemics (retinoids, cyclosporine) or biologics

Is Methotrexate Right for You?

Before starting you on treatment with methotrexate, your doctor might ask several questions, examine you, and discuss with you the benefits and risks. As with any treatment, the risks should not outweigh the benefits.

Your doctor will ask you about other diseases or disorders that could prohibit you from taking methotrexate (e.g., liver and/or kidney disease). Because methotrexate is eliminated by the kidneys, if they do not function properly, the drug cannot be properly removed from the body. In addition, with high doses of methotrexate, there is a possibility of kidney damage, in which case the dose would be lowered or another method of treatment considered.

One of the most significant concerns with long-term use of methotrexate is cirrhosis (scarring) of the liver. In general, it appears that patients at highest risk for cirrhosis are:

• obese
• drinking alcohol while taking methotrexate
• diabetic (the pancreas does not produce enough insulin)
• long-term users of methotrexate

To find out if you have cirrhosis, a liver biopsy might be performed. A liver biopsy involves having a thin needle pass through the skin into the liver to obtain a small piece of tissue, which is then examined to determine if there is any scarring present. A liver biopsy is performed before or shortly after starting methotrexate and then again after several years of long-term use.

Before starting treatment, certain blood tests will also be performed to test the liver, kidneys, and blood cell counts. These tests are usually repeated weekly for one month at the beginning of treatment and if and when the dose of methotrexate is increased. After this, testing will be done regularly. Regular blood work is important because it may help in the early detection of any signs of injury or irritation to your kidneys, liver, or blood cells, and gives your doctor the opportunity to alter your dosage or discontinue the treatment, if necessary.

How Do You Take Methotrexate?
Methotrexate is available in tablets (2.5 milligrams) or as a

liquid that is injected into the muscle. Your doctor will ask you to take methotrexate only once a week.

Taking Medication
- Many medications are taken daily, but it is important that you take methotrexate only once a week (not daily) as prescribed by your doctor.
- Always take only the dosage your doctor prescribed.
- If you miss a dose, take it as soon as possible.
- Because your doctor might change your dose, check the label every time you fill your prescription.
- If you develop severe difficulty breathing or shortness of breath, stop this medication and contact your doctor.
- Notify your doctor immediately if you have taken more medication than prescribed.
- Methotrexate should be kept and stored away from children.

Who Should Not Take Methotrexate?
Patients on methotrexate should not take an antibiotic called trimethoprim sulfamethoxazole (Septra®, Cotrima®, Bactrim®). Also, those who cannot have blood tests done, take medications regularly, or are pregnant (or planning a pregnancy) should not take methotrexate. Other reasons you should not take methotrexate, and drugs that interact with it, are listed below.

Reasons a Psoriasis Patient Should Not Take Methotrexate
- pregnant or nursing
- kidney disease
- liver disease (including a history of)
- immunodeficiency (HIV/AIDS or other)
- active or recurring infections

- stomach ulcer
- current drug or alcohol abuse

*Drugs That Interact with Methotrexate**

- trimethoprim sulfamethoxazole
- nonsteroidal anti-inflammatories drugs (NSAIDs)
- barbiturates (depressants such as pentobarbital sodium)
- triamterene (Dyrenium®) (diuretic)
- pyrimethamine (Daraprim®) (anti-protozoa drug)
- Aspirin®
- penicillin

*This is not a complete list of medications that interact with methotrexate. You should consult with your doctor before taking any new medication, and inform him or her of all medications you are on *before* starting methotrexate.

Side Effects

There are side effects that can develop right away (acute or short-term side effects) or that might appear after a longer period of time (chronic or long-term side effects). If you do experience any side effects, be sure to tell your doctor. Some of the most common side effects of methotrexate are listed in the table on page 127.

What Tests and Follow-ups Are Required While Taking Methotrexate?

Once methotrexate is started, regular follow-up visits are necessary so your doctor can properly monitor both your health and response to treatment. The results of monitoring and testing enable your doctor to modify your dosage in case you need to increase it to improve the results, decrease it to reduce any side effects, or discontinue it altogether.

Side Effects of Methotrexate (MTX)	What You Can Do
Common Side Effects • Loss of appetite or weight • Nausea • Anemia • Fatigue	• These are very common. If they are severe, contact your doctor. • Nausea can be helped by drinking milk or eating something when taking the drug. Folic acid (5 milligrams/day) can also help nausea/vomiting. • Some of these effects can also be managed by reducing the dose or changing the dosing method (e.g., changing from pills to intramuscular injection).
Other Short-Term Side Effects • Mouth blistering • Sun sensitivity • Vomiting • Symptoms of infection (sore throat, fever, cough) • Headache • Easy bruising • Diarrhea	• These are less common, but if they persist for several hours and are severe, contact your doctor immediately. • May cause mouth sores because the dose is too high. • Wear sunscreen and sun protection when going outside. Use precaution when receiving PUVA or UVB. Avoid sun during peak exposure (10 a.m.–2 p.m.). • Folic acid (5 milligrams/day) can help nausea/vomiting. • Contact your doctor • Contact your doctor • Contact your doctor • Contact your doctor
Long-Term Side Effects • Cirrhosis of the liver • Pulmonary toxicity (lungs) • Renal toxicity (kidneys) • Damage to your bone marrow.	• Any of these side effects can occur with prolonged use of MTX. • Your doctor will check to see if you have developed any of these side effects. If they occur, MTX may be reduced or stopped

Cyclosporine

Cyclosporine is a pill given to patients with moderate to severe psoriasis. Initially discovered in 1976, and used as an immune-suppressing drug for organ transplant patients, cyclosporine was observed to also have a beneficial effect on a series of patients who had psoriasis but who were taking the drug for an unrelated disease.

How Does Cyclosporine Work?

Cyclosporine is prescribed for the treatment of severe, resistant, plaque-type psoriasis. Many patients will use cyclosporine after they have failed topical therapies (creams and ointments), ultraviolet therapy (phototherapy), or other oral medications (methotrexate, retinoids). Cyclosporine works by inhibiting the activation of the T-lymphocyte, which is one of the key immune cells responsible for the development of psoriasis. It is highly effective in treating psoriasis, and works rapidly.

Patients Who May Benefit from Cyclosporine
- those with moderate to severe psoriasis who have failed to respond to phototherapy, or other systemic or biologic therapies
- those needing treatment for a psoriasis flare-up
- those who cannot tolerate or have contraindications to other systemic treatments

How Do You Take Cyclosporine?
The medication is generally taken by mouth once daily and the dosage is based on your weight. The starting dose can begin at 2.5 milligrams per kilogram of body weight per day, and can be increased to 5 milligrams/kilogram/day. For example, for a patient weighing 132 pounds (60 kilograms), a starting dose could be 150 milligrams per day. The medication is taken daily and it is important not to miss any doses. If you miss a dose, take it as soon as possible.

Before taking cyclosporine, make sure you read the prescription label carefully. Also be sure to take the exact amount of medicine prescribed by your doctor. Your dose depends on several factors, including the type of psoriasis you have. Your doctor may change your prescribed dose, so it is important to check the label every time you fill your prescription.

Cyclosporine works quite quickly to improve psoriasis compared to methotrexate and retinoids. You could begin to experience improvement in the first few weeks of treatment and, within the first four to eight weeks, the clearing of large areas of psoriasis is not uncommon. However, once treatment with cyclosporine is discontinued, psoriasis will, in all likelihood, recur over several weeks to months. For this reason, it is important that the medication not be stopped abruptly as psoriasis can flare up quickly. Before you stop taking this medication, discuss this step with your doctor as she or he will want to either taper the medication by gradually decreasing the dosage or substitute another treatment. It is also important to understand that cyclosporine is usually discontinued after a year as it can cause kidney damage.

Is Cyclosporine Right for You?

Before beginning treatment with cyclosporine, your doctor will ask you several questions, examine you, and then discuss the possible treatments and their side effects. If you and your doctor decide cyclosporine is a good choice for you, some tests will be performed, including a careful skin and physical examination, a test of your kidney function, and a complete blood cell count. In addition, your blood pressure will be measured prior to starting the medication and regularly thereafter.

Who Should Not Take Cyclosporine?

Cyclosporine might not be a good choice for you if you have kidneys that are not functioning normally, if you have uncontrolled high blood pressure, or if you have an allergy to the drug.

Reasons a Psoriasis Patient Should Not Take Cyclosporine
- decreased kidney function
- uncontrolled high blood pressure (hypertension)
- allergy to cyclosporine
- receiving live vaccinations
- taking medications that interact with cyclosporine

- active infection
- immunodeficiency (HIV/AIDS or other)
- receiving other immunosuppressive agents
- pregnant or nursing
- unable to attend regular doctor visits or have blood tests taken to monitor for side effects

*Drugs and Supplements That Interact with Cyclosporine**
- nonsteroidal anti-inflammatory drugs
- antibiotics (erythromycin [Eryc®], clarithromycin [Biaxin®], azithromycin [Zithromax®], doxycycline [Vibra-Tabs®])
- trimethoprim sulfamethoxazole (Septra®)
- immunosuppressive drugs (tacrolimus [Prograf®], melphalan [Alkeran®])
- oral contraceptives
- warfarin
- St.-John's-wort
- grapefruit, grapefruit juice

*This is not a complete list of the medications that interact with cyclosporine. Consult with your doctor or pharmacist before taking any medication.

Side Effects
Cyclosporine suppresses the immune system (immunosuppressant), and there are possible side effects that are mainly related to immunosuppression. In addition, kidney toxicity, high blood pressure, and potential interaction with other drugs are other risks. Cyclosporine's risks and benefits should be carefully considered before starting the treatment. Side effects are usually reversible if treatment with cyclosporine is stopped.

Common Side Effects of Cyclosporine
- abnormal functioning of the kidney
- high blood pressure (hypertension)
- tremor
- headache
- numbness, tingling
- excessive growth of hair (hypertrichosis)
- swelling of the gums in the mouth
- nausea, abdominal pain
- diarrhea
- muscle pain
- joint pain
- increased blood potassium levels
- increased blood plasma levels of cholesterol, fats
- increased risk of cancer

There are also some less common but serious side effects that are important to recognize. Many patients are concerned by the reported increased risk of cancer with cyclosporine. For example, lymphoma has been reported in some patients taking cyclosporine. Lymphoma is most commonly seen in patients taking higher doses of medication, and has been reported in those who are also on other immunosuppressant medications. It is not clear if cyclosporine is entirely responsible for the increased risk of lymphoma as these other drugs could also play a role. In addition, certain studies have shown that patients with psoriasis may have an increased risk of lymphoma in general.

An increased risk of skin cancers has also been reported in patients taking cyclosporine, many of whom might have received phototherapy prior to using cyclosporine, thereby increasing the risk of skin cancer. The most common types of skin cancers in patients receiving cyclosporine therapy are squamous cell carcinoma and basal cell carcinoma. Fortunately, both these cancers are highly curable, particularly when detected early. Consequently, if you notice a changing area on your skin or an area that is not healing, report it to your doctor immediately so that the lesion can be checked and, if necessary, removed. Although there are reasons why a patient taking cyclosporines might develop lymphoma, it is important to recognize that medications that affect the immune system might play a role in the development of such cancers.

What Tests or Follow-ups Are Required While on Cyclosporine?

Your blood pressure will be measured prior to starting cyclosporine, then regularly during the initial and subsequent months of therapy. Blood pressure will be carefully monitored because high blood pressure is one of the side effects of this medication. Blood tests measuring how your kidneys are working will also be performed. This test works by measuring your creatinine, a waste product found in urine. A 25 percent increase from normal blood levels of creatinine can indicate mild kidney damage. This is generally reversible when the dosage is decreased or cyclosporine therapy is discontinued. In addition, other blood tests, such as cholesterol and potassium, might be tested at the same time as the kidney tests are taken. Before you start on any other medications, consult your doctor.

Oral Retinoids

Retinoids are synthetic drugs derived from vitamin A. There are two types of retinoids used in dermatology: isotretinoin (Accutane®) and acitretin (Soriatane®). Isotretinoin contains an ingredient related to vitamin A and is used mainly to treat acne. Acitretin is also related to vitamin A, but is prescribed by dermatologists to treat psoriasis. Another type of retinoid that is still in clinical research trials is oral tazarotene, which is the systemic form of topical tazarotene used occasionally for treating localized psoriasis (see Chapter 9).

Acitretin (Soriatane®)

Before you take acitretin tell your doctor if you are:
- pregnant or planning a pregnancy
- taking vitamins or other supplements containing vitamin A
- sensitive to retinoids
- allergic to any food or drugs
- taking any other drugs
- taking an antibiotic (particularly tetracycline [Sumycin®])

Acitretin is used to treat moderate to severe psoriasis that has failed to respond to topical therapies. It is particularly effective for erythrodermic, palmoplantar, and pustular psoriasis (see Chapter 1). When used to treat severe plaque-type psoriasis, patients might experience only a partial improvement, and it can take several months to see any improvement. You might notice a temporary worsening of your condition in the first month of use. In this case, your dose of acitretin might be increased or used in combination with other treatments, such as topical corticosteroids, calcipotriol, or phototherapy (see Chapters 9 and 10).

How Does Acitretin Work?

In psoriasis, the skin cell turnover is accelerated from the normal twenty to thirty days for a cell to mature from the basal layer to be shed, to three to four days (see Chapter 1). Acitretin helps to slow that rapid growth and, as a result, it reduces the scaling, redness, and thickness seen in the skin of certain psoriasis patients.

How Do You Take Acitretin?

This medication is available in soft gelatin capsules (10 and 25 milligram strengths) and is usually taken once daily with food or just after a meal. For adults, a starting dose of 25–50 milligrams per day is usually prescribed. The dose may be increased after about four to eight weeks to 50–75 milligrams/day to improve the response. If you miss a dose, take it as soon as possible. Do not double your doses.

Before taking acitretin, read the prescription label carefully. Also be sure to take the exact amount of medicine prescribed by your doctor. Your dose depends on several factors, including the type of psoriasis you have. Your doctor may change your prescribed dose so it is important to check the label every time you fill your prescription.

Is Acitretin Right for You?

Before beginning treatment with acitretin, your doctor may ask you several questions, examine you, and discuss with you the different treatments available, side effects, and reasons that some patients should not take acitretin. Some tests will also be performed, including a pregnancy test (in fertile women), a complete blood cell count, and liver and kidney function tests. In addition, a blood lipid (fat) test will be done (you will not be able to eat for 12 hours prior to the test). Blood lipid tests include testing triglycerides and cholesterol levels.

Acitretin is well known to cause birth defects when given to pregnant women. Those who are fertile should use two effective forms of birth control for at least one month before starting acitretin, and a pregnancy test should be done one week prior to beginning treatment, which should be on day two or three of your menstrual period. In women of childbearing potential, alcohol should not be consumed during therapy or for two months after therapy is stopped. Also, it is very important that effective birth control is continued for at least two years after stopping acitretin. No one who is taking acitretin can donate blood—if a pregnant woman was to receive blood from a person on acitretin, the unborn fetus could be seriously harmed.

> ### Retinoids and Birth Defects
>
> All retinoids can cause severe birth defects in the developing fetus. Therefore, it is critical that women who are pregnant or who could become pregnant during therapy or for two years after treatment do not take acitretin. Females who could become pregnant should continue birth control for up to two years after stopping acitretin.

Who Should Not Take Acitretin?

Women of childbearing potential must not drink alcohol during therapy and for two months after therapy is stopped. If alcohol is consumed, acitretin can change inside the patient's body to a form of the drug that can remain in the body for an extended period of time. This conversion increases the risk of birth defects if a woman was to become pregnant after stopping acitretin. Women of childbearing potential should not use acitretin unless they are willing to use reliable birth control while taking the medication and for at least two years after treatment is stopped.

Before starting acitretin treatment it is also important to consult your doctor if you are taking any medication or supplement, especially vitamin A, tetracyclines, methotrexate, or supplements such as St. John's Wort. These could increase your risk of side effects.

Do not have surgical cosmetic procedures on your skin while taking acitretin because retinoids can increase your chance of scarring or inflammation. Avoid such procedures or avoid oral retinoids for up to six months before having such procedures.

As well, you should protect yourself from the sun and avoid using tanning beds. Some patients can expose themselves to ultraviolet radiation (UVB/PUVA) if under a doctor's supervision. Retinoids are known to increase your skin's sensitivity to ultraviolet light in both natural and artificial sunlight.

Sun Safety Tips
- Avoid peak sun exposure when the sun's rays are strongest (between 10 a.m. and 3 p.m.).
- Seek the shade.
- Use a broad-spectrum sunscreen with an SPF of at least 15 that protects against both UVA and UVB.
- Wear protective clothing, particularly a broad-brimmed hat and long sleeves.

Reasons a Psoriasis Patient Should Not Take Acitretin
- pregnant or planning to become pregnant
- nursing women
- unwilling to use birth control
- experience an abnormal decrease in the number of white blood cells (leukopenia)
- experiencing moderate to severe elevation of cholesterol or triglycerides
- experiencing major liver abnormality
- experiencing major kidney abnormality

Drugs and Supplements That Interact with Acitretin*
- vitamin A or any other supplement containing vitamin A that exceeds the minimum recommended allowance
- certain antibiotics (minocycline (Minocin®), doxycycline (Vibra-Tabs®), tetracycline)
- cyclosporine
- alcohol

- methotrexate
- St.-John's-wort

*This is not a complete list of medications that interact with acitretin. You should consult with your doctor before taking any new medication.

Side Effects

While there are many potential side effects with acitretin, most are mild and short-lived. Acitretin has a better safety profile than most other available systemic agents, and is a useful medication for appropriate psoriasis patients.

Some side effects occur after a few weeks of starting treatment, but will often improve. These include chapped lips, dry skin, nosebleeds, dry mouth, dry or irritated eyes, and peeling of the skin of the fingertips, palms, and soles. Hair loss is not common, but can be very distressing for those affected; however, hair will gradually regrow after treatment ceases. If you experience joint and muscle pain, it is wise to avoid excessive exercising, particularly weight lifting and contact sports. Other adverse effects are less frequent, but can be more serious.

Increased pressure behind the eye is relatively uncommon, but can occur with acitretin use. The risk of developing this condition (pseudotumor cerebri) is increased in young, overweight women. Common symptoms include severe headache, nausea, vomiting, and blurred vision. If these symptoms occur, immediately contact your doctor, who might discontinue the treatment.

Although rare, depression and suicide have been reported, mostly in association with isotretinoin; however, there is insufficient information to indicate that retinoids such as isotretinoin or acitretin *cause* depression. Several studies based on drug-use registries in Saskatchewan and the United

Kingdom showed no increase in suicide or depression with acitretin, compared to people who were not taking this medication. Still, it is important to be aware of this association, and to pay close attention to any changes in mood and any symptoms of depression. If you happen to experience feelings of sadness, irritability, fatigue, difficulty concentrating, or loss of appetite, you should immediately contact your doctor. Other rare side effects include injury to the liver, increase in blood lipids, and inflammation of the pancreas (pancreatitis).

Side Effects of Acitretin

What May Happen	What You Can Do
Skin Side Effects	
dry skin (xerosis)	• use a moisturizer or emollient
scaly, itchy skin	• use a moisturizer or emollient
increased sun sensitivity	• wear sunscreen/protective clothes
skin peeling (palms, soles, and fingertips)	• apply a moisturizer; if severe, contact your doctor
Hair Side Effects	
temporary hair loss	• contact your doctor, who may discontinue therapy
Eye Side Effects	
dry eyes	• use an artificial tear product
abnormal sensitivity to light (photophobia)	• wear sunglasses to protect your eyes
increased pressure behind the eyes	• if you have severe headaches, nausea, vomiting, or (pseudotumor cerebri) blurred vision, stop the medication and contact your doctor
Mouth Side Effects	
chapped lips	• apply an ointment
bleeding gums	• see your doctor
Nose Side Effects	For all:
dry nose	• apply nasal lubricants
runny nose	• use a humidifier
nosebleeds	
Other	
joint pain and muscle pain	• decrease exercise; take an anti-inflammatory; if severe, contact your doctor
birth defects	• do not take acitretin if you are pregnant, plan to be pregnant, or are nursing

Once acitretin therapy is started, regular follow-up visits are necessary to monitor your response to the medication, and to determine if you have any side effects from the medication. Your doctor will be able to increase your dosage if the results need to be improved, decrease it to reduce any side effects, or discontinue it altogether.

What Tests or Follow-ups Are Required While on Acitretin?
Regular blood tests will be completed while patients are on acitretin to monitor the blood cell count, liver and kidney function, and to ensure that female patients of childbearing age do not get pregnant. Also, the triglyceride and cholesterol levels will be tested, so fasting will be required for 12 hours prior to testing.

Stop taking acitretin and contact your doctor immediately if you become pregnant while on this medication or within two years after stopping this medication.

TWELVE

Biologic Therapies

An exciting and rapidly advancing area in the treatment of psoriasis and psoriatic arthritis involves the use of a new class of medications called biologic agents. These are highly targeted medications developed to focus on key steps that lead to the development of psoriasis lesions. One of the important advances in understanding the causes of psoriasis is that imbalances in the immune system send faulty messages to the skin and cause the raised, red, scaly lesions of psoriasis. The new understandings have allowed biotechnology companies to develop these new biologic drugs to target such abnormalities in the immune system. As with all new therapies, the long-term side effects of these drugs are unknown. You must always keep this in mind. Your doctor will help you understand the risks and benefits of treatment for your particular case. Biologic agents are significantly different from traditional or conventional medications in several ways:

1. Biologics are often naturally occurring substances. Traditional medications are made by mixing chemicals to form liquids or pills. Biologics are different because they are made from living cells, such as viruses, animal cells, and human cells. Biologic drugs have natural counterparts, such as proteins, enzymes, antibodies, or nucleic acids (e.g., DNA). An example of a biologic drug used in another disease is insulin (used to control diabetes).

2. Biologics are so-called "designer" drugs. Traditional drugs have not been specifically developed for the treatment of psoriasis. For example, cyclosporine (Sandimmune®) was initially developed as an organ transplantation drug and was found by chance to work for psoriasis while treating patients for a different condition. By contrast, biologic molecules are custom-made, using a technique called recombinant technology, to target key abnormalities in the immune system that result in the red, scaly, raised skin of psoriasis and the tender, swollen joints of psoriatic arthritis. By specifically targeting key steps in the immune system, biologics are able to correct imbalances in the immune system and therefore improve psoriasis. While existing therapies such as cyclosporine and methotrexate (Rheumatrex®) also target the immune system, the new therapies are much more specific in correcting the imbalance of the immune response in psoriasis. It is hoped that this specific, targeted action will result in safer and effective new drugs.

3. Biologic drugs are given in a different manner than traditional drugs. Traditional drugs are usually delivered by mouth. Biologic drugs are usually made of proteins and cannot be taken orally because the digestion process would destroy them. Instead, biologics are given by injection under the skin, into the muscle or by intravenous infusion.

4. Biologic drugs may be more effective than traditional drugs. Recent research has shown that certain biologic drugs (adalimumab, infliximab) were more effective than methotrexate in a short-term randomized controlled study.

5. Biologic drugs are very expensive. Biologic drugs are complicated molecules that are difficult to make. The agents go through extensive testing to prove they are safe and effective. Partly for these reasons, biologic drugs tend to be costly.

How Do Biologics Work?

As outlined in Chapter 3, activated T-cells can travel to the surface of the skin and start an inflammatory reaction in which skin cells multiply much faster than normal, resulting in the formation of psoriatic plaques. Biologic drugs work by interfering with specific components of the autoimmune response and can target those chemicals involved in causing psoriasis.

Alefacept (a-LEH-fa-sep-t) (Amevive®)
Alefacept is a fully human biologic agent that targets the activated T-cells, which are believed to cause the skin lesions of psoriasis. It prevents the T-cells from becoming overactive and reduces the number of activated T-cells in your body. It is the first biologic agent approved in Canada and the United States for the treatment of psoriasis.

How Alefacept Works
Alefacept reduces the number of activated T-cells in the body's circulation and in the skin, thereby inhibiting the release of the chemicals (cytokines) that are partly responsible for causing the lesions of psoriasis. In doing so, alefacept can inhibit key steps in the overactive immune system that results in psoriasis.

How Is Alefacept Given?
Usually, alefacept is either administered at your doctor's office or at home by a nurse or it can be self-administered (after you have had appropriate training from your doctor or nurse) as a single injection into the muscle, or just under the skin, once a week for twelve weeks. Alefacept may be recommended to be used for sixteen weeks in certain patients. A blood sample is also taken on a regular basis to monitor your T-cells while on alefacept.

1. Before you start alefacept: You and your doctor will review

the risks, benefits, and alternatives to alefacept. Your doctor might give you an informed consent form outlining these risks and benefits. You are entitled to review this document on your own, and with your doctor or nurse, and sign it. This document is intended to give you an additional opportunity to review the risks, benefits, and alternatives. Also, you will need some blood work done prior to starting alefacept.

2. Starting treatment with alefacept: The medication is administered by intramuscular injection. In the U.S., it is given at your doctor's office or at home by a nurse. In Canada, it can be self-administered. If you and your doctor decide that self-injection is appropriate, you will be given training by a health care professional. This training will give you information on how to prepare the drug for injection and show you the proper method for giving yourself an intramuscular injection. You should not try to inject yourself until this training has been given and you are comfortable with the process. The makers of alefacept have developed a comprehensive support program that provides a variety of services.

What Results Can You Expect from Alefacept?

With alefacept, improvements are not usually immediate but occur over several months. Many patients will continue to exhibit improvement even after the last dose of a twelve-week course. Combination therapy, such as topical steroids or phototherapy or other systemic medications (e.g., retinoids), can also be used to improve speed of onset of clearance of psoriasis.

An interesting finding in early studies with alefacept was that by reducing the number of T-cells in circulation and in the skin of patients with psoriasis, prolonged psoriasis-free periods could be attained (remission). On average, a patient who has responded well to alefacept can have a significant improvement in psoriasis that can last up to eight months or longer.

In clinical research studies, an excellent level of improvement (75 percent improvement in the score of the Psoriasis Area and Severity Index [PASI]) was seen in about 21 percent of patients, and a good response was seen in 42 percent of patients (a good response is defined as a 50 percent improvement in the PASI score) two weeks after stopping therapy. Because improvements continue after treatment is stopped, response rates can be higher than those listed above, which are at two weeks after stopping therapy. Based on the overall response rate, 33 percent of patients had an excellent level of improvement and 57 percent had a good level of improvement. After a second twelve-week course, 43 percent had an excellent level of improvement and 69 percent had a good level. Additional courses showed further improvement.

One of the unique aspects of alefacept therapy is that the onset of activity is slower than that of many other medications. The positive results, however, can last for up to a year or longer in certain patients, which is a unique and valuable part of this therapy. In general, patients can expect to receive a response within two to three months after beginning therapy.

If alefacept is your only therapy, be patient and try not to get frustrated—remember that it could be months before you see an improvement. However, some patients will see an improvement after several weeks. Many doctors will add topical steroids or other therapies to accelerate the onset of improvement. There have been studies combining ultraviolet light therapy (phototherapy) with alefacept, and many patients have had a speedier improvement. This combination of therapies was found to be tolerable and safe in the short-term.

After the first twelve-week course, your doctor will decide if a second course is right for you. Alefacept is currently being studied for treatment of psoriatic arthritis and has demonstrated significant improvements.

What You Should Tell the Doctor before Starting Alefacept
Alefacept can both affect your normal immune response and make you more susceptible to infections. You should tell your doctor about any other health problems you have now or have had in the past. If any of the following conditions apply, tell your doctor before you start alefacept therapy:
- are pregnant or are planning to become pregnant
- are breast-feeding
- have had a recent severe infection or are prone to chronic or recurring infections
- have, have had, or have been exposed to tuberculosis
- have a history of immune suppression (such as HIV/AIDS)
- have a history of cancer
- have a history of allergy to alefacept
- are taking any other medications, especially immunosuppressive agents or herbal supplements

Who Should Not Take Alefacept?
- those with a T-cell count lower than 250 cells/microliter
- those who are pregnant or breast-feeding
- those who have a serious infection, or frequent recurrence of serious infections
- those who have HIV/AIDS
- those who have cancer (with the exception of certain types of skin cancer that have been treated)
- those who are allergic to alefacept or any of its components

What You Should Tell the Doctor While Taking Alefacept
As always, it is important to follow your doctor's instructions, keep your appointments for injections, and obtain all blood work as directed by your doctor. If you develop any of the following conditions while taking alefacept, immediately contact your doctor.

You experience a decrease in your T-lymphocyte number: A decrease in the number of T-lymphocytes (one of the types of white blood cells measured during a complete blood count) is called lymphopenia. If your T-lymphocytes drop below a certain number while on alefacept, your doctor will stop your treatment until they increase (levels of CD4+ T-lymphocyte cells should be greater than 250 cells/microliter). If these levels are below normal prior to starting alefacept treatment, you should not start until your cell count is normal or above normal. Your doctor will determine this before starting therapy. It is important to get your blood work done regularly while on alefacept as directed by your doctor.

You develop an infection: If you develop an infection or symptoms of an infection, you should contact your doctor. If the infection is mild, it may not be necessary for you to stop treatment. However, certain infections may require you to do so. Symptoms can include fever, fatigue, and/or a cough. Other symptoms could include a raised, hot, red area of skin that is spreading. If you feel unwell but do not have a fever, it is still important to tell your doctor. Since alefacept can suppress your immune system, your body may not respond to an infection with a fever as it would normally. If you develop a serious infection alefacept should be stopped until it is fully treated. Any medication that your doctor prescribes for the treatment of infections should be taken immediately.

You develop cancer (malignancies): If you develop cancer while taking alefacept, tell your doctor right away. Alefacept is an immunosuppressant and has a potential to increase your risk of cancer. Alefacept reduces the number of T-cells, which are important in fighting and preventing serious infections and cancer. The role of alefacept in the development of cancer is unknown. In clinical trials, the incidence of cancer in patients treated with alefacept was low and similar to those taking a placebo. Long-term follow-up studies are required to determine the safety of this medication.

You become pregnant: If you become pregnant while taking alefacept, contact your doctor immediately. In the United States, there is a pregnancy registry that you can enroll in by calling 1-866-263-8483.

You need to receive a vaccine: The efficacy and safety of live vaccines administered while a patient is taking alefacept is not known.

What Side Effects Can Alefacept Cause?
Side effects are possible with any medication, including biologic agents; however, clinical studies have shown that alefacept is well tolerated. There is no evidence of psoriasis rapidly recurring (rebound) after stopping therapy. The most common side effects, experienced by more than 5 percent of patients, were:
- sore throat
- runny nose
- nausea
- fatigue
- diarrhea
- itch
- headaches
- pain, swelling, and redness at the site of injection

Alefacept is an immunosuppressant and has the potential to increase your risk of cancer. The role of alefacept in the development of cancer is unknown. In clinical trials, the incidence of cancer in patients treated with alefacept was low and similar to those taking a placebo.

How Do You Store Alefacept?

When alefacept is administered at your doctor's office, it will usually be provided when you come to the clinic. If a nurse comes to your home and administers the injection, you may have to store the medication.

- Do not use the medicine after the expiry date on either the vial of alefacept or the water used for injection. Do not use after the last day of the last month stamped on either vial.
- The dose pack should be stored in the refrigerator between 36°–45°F (2°–8°C).
- If there is not enough room in the refrigerator for the entire dose pack (a vial of dilutant, syringe, needles, bandage, alcohol pack, and gauze pads), it is important that the vial of alefacept is refrigerated. Other parts of the dose pack can be stored at room temperature.
- You might want to take the alefacept out of the refrigerator 30 minutes before you inject, which will allow the medication to warm to room temperature and will be more comfortable for you to inject.
- Once you mix the dilutant with the alefacept, use it immediately.
- If necessary, you can keep the mixed solution in the refrigerator for up to 4 hours. If you don't use it within 4 hours, dispose of the solution.

Tumor Necrosis Factor-Alpha

People with psoriasis and psoriatic arthritis can produce increased amounts of an important protein (cytokine) known as tumor necrosis factor-alpha or TNF-alpha, which can cause the red, scaly, raised areas of the skin and tender, swollen joints.

TNF-alpha is found in higher than normal amounts in the affected skin and joints and can trigger inflammation in these areas. Blocking this inflammatory messenger can reduce inflammation of the joints in psoriatic arthritis, and prevent and treat the appearance of skin lesions in psoriasis.

Three biologic agents, etanercept (Enbrel®), adalimumab (Humira®), and infliximab (Remicade®), block TNF-alpha and are currently approved in the United States and Canada for the treatment of psoriatic arthritis and psoriasis. These agents can neutralize the undesirable inflammatory effects of TNF-alpha in the skin and joints.

Infliximab (in-fliks-ih-MAB) (Remicade®)

Infliximab is a biologic drug that binds and blocks TNF-alpha. As noted earlier, biologic drugs are made from living cells, such as viruses, animal cells, and human cells. A small portion of infliximab is derived from mice. Infliximab is a very selective agent that localizes at the site of inflammation in the skin and blood vessel walls. It is able to kill cells that have TNF-alpha on their surfaces and acts like a sponge, soaking up TNF-alpha and removing it from the body's circulation.

How Is Infliximab Given?

The drug is given by intravenous infusion over about a 2-hour period. It is administered by a trained health care professional either in a private clinic or in a hospital.

There are four steps to the infusion process.

1. Before you start infliximab: Your doctor will review with you the risks, benefits, side effects, and alternatives. Your doctor might give you an informed consent form outlining these risks and benefits. You are entitled to review this document on your own, and with your doctor or nurse, and sign it if you are comfortable with what you have read,

heard, and discussed with your health care providers. The intention is to give you an additional opportunity to review the risks, benefits, and alternatives before you start treatment. You will need some blood work done, a tuberculosis skin test, and possibly a chest X-ray prior to starting the medication.

Infliximab: Key Points

- biologic agent that targets the TNF-alpha cytokine
- given by intravenous infusion over approximately 2 hours
- patients receive infusions initially and then at weeks two, six, and ten
- after those infusions, patients may be infused every eight weeks to maintain improvements
- very rapid onset of action
- most patients respond to therapy

---

2. Day of the infusion: When you arrive at the infusion clinic or hospital, a nurse will check all your vital signs, such as temperature, blood pressure, and heart rate, before administering infliximab.

3. Infusion: You will sit in a chair and a trained professional will insert a small needle into your arm. This may create a slight pinching sensation, which is only temporary. A small narrow tube called a catheter will replace the needle. The medication travels from a small bag through tubing into the catheter and into your arm. It is important not to make any sudden movements or the catheter may be dislodged from your arm.

4. During the infusion: Your nurse will regularly monitor your progress, check your vital signs, and ensure you are tolerating the therapy well. During this time, you can relax, read or, in some clinics, watch television. If you develop any of the following, you should notify your doctor or nurse immediately: hives/rash; wheezing or tightness in

your chest; or swelling of your eyelids, face, or lips. If you develop such symptoms, your doctor or nurse may stop the infusion and administer another counteracting medication through an intravenous line or under the surface of your skin, or you may be asked to take a medication by mouth.

You will be monitored for 1–2 hours after the infusion.

What Results Can You Expect from Infliximab?

Well-designed clinical studies have evaluated the effects of infliximab in psoriasis and psoriatic arthritis. Infliximab is one of the most effective, if not the most effective, medications in treating psoriasis, with a rapid onset of action. Approximately 80 percent of patients in the 5 milligram/kilogram dosing group had an excellent response to infliximab. In addition, the response to infliximab was very rapid, having a significant effect within four weeks for many patients.

Several distinguishing features of infliximab have become evident from these studies:

- Infliximab patients experience a rapid improvement in psoriasis.
- Improvements are seen as early as two weeks after an infliximab infusion.
- A significant improvement was noted, with more than 80 percent of patients achieving an excellent improvement.

What You Should Tell the Doctor before Starting Infliximab

You should tell your doctor if you:

- are pregnant or planning on becoming pregnant
- are breast-feeding
- have a history of heart failure
- have problems with your immune system (HIV/AIDS)

- have had a recent severe infection or are prone to chronic or recurring infections
- have, have had, or have been exposed to tuberculosis; you will need to have a tuberculosis skin test done; if you have tuberculosis, you will need medication to treat the tuberculosis before you start infliximab therapy in order to prevent a recurrence of tuberculosis infections
- are taking any medications or herbal supplements
- have had an allergic reaction to infliximab or one of its components
- have a history of liver disease (i.e., hepatitis B)
- have problems or diseases with the nervous system such as multiple sclerosis; if you experience any numbness, tingling, or visual changes before, during, or after infliximab treatment, you should tell your doctor; a small number of patients who have received infliximab have experienced a worsening of their multiple sclerosis and other rare diseases of the nervous system (Guillain-Barré, optic neuritis)

Who Should Not Take Infliximab?

Who should not take Infliximab (Remicade®)?	Why
• If you are pregnant or planning on becoming pregnant	• Safety not established as of yet
• If you are breast-feeding	• Safety not established as of yet
• If you have severe heart failure	• Patients with severe heart failure had worsening of their heart failure while on infliximab
• If you have tuberculosis	• Infliximab suppresses TNF-alpha and can lead to recurrence of tuberculosis
• If you have any history of recurrent, recent severe, or current infections	• TNF-alpha suppresses the immune system, which is important in fighting infections
• If you have multiple sclerosis	• Could worsen multiple sclerosis
• If you have a history of liver disease (hepatitis B)	• Could worsen hepatitis

What You Should Tell the Doctor While Taking Infliximab
Contact your doctor while taking infliximab if any of the following occur:

You develop an allergic reaction: Some patients can develop an allergic reaction to biologic agents, which are produced from living cells. Infliximab is partly developed from mouse cells. Your body might recognize infliximab as a foreign substance, so it is possible to develop a reaction to the drug. This reaction can be mild and might present as an itch or hives. Serious allergic reactions are less common but are possible. These include difficulty breathing, wheezing, hives, and high or low blood pressure. Tell your doctor immediately if you develop any of these signs or symptoms during or after treatment so that she or he can reduce the speed of the infusion, stop the infusion, and/or prescribe medications. If you have a very severe reaction, your doctor will stop infliximab treatment altogether.

Some reactions can occur several days to one week after infliximab infusion. These delayed reactions can involve muscle or joint paint, fever, or a rash. Tell your doctor if you develop any of these symptoms.

You develop an infection: As with other treatments, it is very important to advise your doctor if you develop an infection or any symptoms of an infection. If your doctor gives you treatment for an infection, it should be taken right away and as prescribed. Treatment with infliximab should be stopped if you develop a serious infection. Symptoms could include fever, tiredness, cough, and flu-like symptoms. If you feel unwell but do not have a fever, it is still important to tell your doctor. Since infliximab suppresses your immune system, your body may not respond to an infection with a fever as it would normally. Medications that suppress your immune system make you more susceptible to developing an infection.

If your doctor gives you treatment for an infection, it should be taken right away and as prescribed. The treatment with infliximab should be stopped if you develop a serious infection.

After your infection has been treated, it is usually possible to have infliximab again to treat your psoriasis.

You develop the symptoms of heart failure: Tell your doctor immediately if you develop new or worsening symptoms of heart failure such as shortness of breath or swelling of your feet, ankles, or calves.

Your body weight changes: The amount of infliximab is based on your weight. If your body weight changes significantly, your doctor might change your dose.

You require a vaccine: You should not receive live vaccines while taking infliximab. Tell your doctor if you need a vaccine.

If you develop cancer: Tell your doctor right away. Infliximab can suppress the immune system, which is important in fighting cancer.

What Side Effects Can Infliximab Cause?
Side effects are possible with any medication, including any of the biologic agents. These medications are specifically designed to target a key process in the immune abnormalities of psoriasis. It is hoped that these medications will be safer in the long term for patients partly because of the specific way in which they work. Most of these medications have been monitored only for short-term safety because they are so new. In the future, it will be very important to ensure these medications are safe over the long term. Infliximab has been given to more than 1 million people worldwide since 1998. It has been approved in Canada for the treatment of Crohn's disease and rheumatoid arthritis; approval is pending for treatment of psoriasis in Canada and the United States.

Most of infliximab's side effects are mild and tend to resolve on their own or with additional treatment. However, as with any medication, there are possibilities of less common but severe side effects. Additional side effects are listed below:
- serious infusion reactions such as hives, difficulty breathing, and low blood pressure
- mild infusion reactions such as rash or itchy skin
- upper respiratory infections
- headache
- nausea
- cough
- sinusitis
- infections due to low immune response

Higher rates of lymphoma were reported in patients receiving infliximab. Many of these patients were on other immunosuppressant medications at the time or had been in the past. In addition, they also had other medical conditions, e.g., rheumatoid arthritis. Because these factors could have predisposed these patients to developing lymphoma, it is unclear how and if infliximab will increase a patient's risk of lymphoma.

Cancers, heart failure, liver injury, and neurologic events were rarely reported in patients receiving infliximab. It is not clear how and if infliximab has caused these rare side effects.

Etanercept (ee-tan-NER-sept)
This biologic therapy is currently approved in Canada and the U.S. for the treatment of adolescents with rheumatoid arthritis. It has also been approved for children with juvenile rheumatoid arthritis, and has been studied in children with psoriasis. It is approved in Europe for children aged 8 and up with psoriasis.

Etanercept targets and blocks the inflammatory messenger

TNF-alpha, which is made by cells in the immune system and sends faulty signals to the skin and joints. Patients with psoriasis and psoriatic arthritis produce too much TNF-alpha, which results in inflammation, causing red, scaly skin lesions and swollen, tender joints. Etanercept reduces inflammation by blocking TNF-alpha's inflammatory message and works like a sponge to reduce the amount of TNF-alpha in the skin and joints.

Etanercept works faster than some other drugs, and many patients will notice an improvement within the first month of treatment. In others, it can take up to three months and for a few it might take up to six months before improvement is seen.

How Is Etanercept Given?

Etanercept is given by an injection just under the surface of the skin. Etanercept is not currently approved for psoriasis in Canada, but is approved for psoriatic arthritis. It is self-administered by patients with psoriatic arthritis in one of two ways:

1. Once weekly—two injections of 25 milligrams each on the same day.
2. Twice weekly—one injection of 25 milligrams, given three to four days apart. In clinical studies with psoriasis, etanercept has also been given in this way and been found to work very well. Even better results were obtained when etanercept was given in higher doses (50 milligrams—given as two 25 milligram injections—twice weekly. Another formulation involves one syringe with a single 50 milligram injection). Before you start etanercept, your doctor will review with you the risks, benefits, and alternatives. Your doctor might give you an informed consent form outlining these risks and benefits. You are entitled to review this document on your own, and with your doctor or nurse, and sign it. The intention is to give you additional oppor-

tunity to review the risks, benefits, and alternatives to etanercept before starting the treatment. Also, you will need some blood work done and a tuberculosis skin test prior to starting the medication.

Your doctor or nurse will give you detailed instructions for preparing and giving an injection. There is also an information package provided with your etanercept that will have step-by-step instructions. If you have any questions, ask your doctor or nurse. There is also a toll-free number for assistance and answering questions in the United States and Canada (see "Further Resources," page 188).

What Results Can You Expect from Etanercept?

Clinical studies have been performed using etanercept in psoriasis and psoriatic arthritis. These studies established that etanercept showed excellent improvement in both psoriatic arthritis and psoriasis.

Etanercept was proven to be highly effective in studies to date, with approximately 34 percent of patients on 25 milligrams twice weekly and 49 percent receiving 50 milligrams twice weekly having an excellent response. A good response was experienced by 64 percent of those receiving 25 milligrams twice weekly and 77 percent of those receiving 50 milligrams twice weekly.

As seen with the other biologic agents, continuing to give additional therapy over time can provide an additional improvement. Etanercept has been used in combination with other types of treatment such as methotrexate, NSAIDs, or SAARDs in the treatment of psoriatic arthritis.

What You Should Tell the Doctor before Starting Etanercept
You should tell your doctor if you:
- are pregnant or plan on becoming pregnant
- are breast-feeding
- have problems with your immune system (HIV/AIDS)
- have a history of heart failure
- have a history of cancer
- have tuberculosis, have had it, or have been recently exposed to it; you will need to have a tuberculosis skin test done; if you have tuberculosis, you will need medication to treat the tuberculosis before you start etanercept therapy to prevent worsening of your tuberculosis
- have had a recent severe infection, or are prone to infections or recurring infections
- are taking any other medications or herbal supplements
- have an allergy to etanercept or any of its components
- have problems or diseases with the nervous system such as multiple sclerosis; if you experience any numbness, tingling, or visual changes before, during, or after etanercept treatment, you should tell your doctor; a small number of patients who have received etanercept have experienced a worsening in their multiple sclerosis and other rare diseases of the nervous system (Guillain-Barré, optic neuritis)

What You Should Tell the Doctor While Taking Etanercept
If you develop any of the following while taking etanercept, you should contact your doctor immediately:

Infections: If you develop an infection or symptoms of an infection, you might need to stop taking etanercept; contact your doctor. If your doctor gives you a treatment for an infection, it should be taken right away and as prescribed. Treatment with etanercept should be stopped if you develop a serious infection. Symptoms may include fever, fatigue, and/or a cough. Other symptoms could include a raised, hot, red area of skin that is spreading. If you feel unwell but do not have a fever, it is still important to tell your doctor. Since etanercept can suppress your immune system, your body may not respond to an infection with a fever as it would normally.

If your doctor gives you treatment for an infection, it should be taken right away and as prescribed. The treatment with etanercept should be stopped if you develop a serious infection.

Symptoms of heart failure: Tell your doctor immediately if you develop new or worsening symptoms of heart failure, such as shortness of breath or swelling of your feet, ankles, or calves.

If you develop cancer: Tell your doctor right away. Etanercept can suppress the immune system, which is important in fighting cancer.

Vaccination: You should not receive live vaccines while taking etanercept. Tell your doctor if you need a vaccine.

Who Should Not Take Etanercept?

Who should not take Etanercept (Enbrel®)?	Why
• If you are pregnant or plan on becoming pregnant	• Safety not established as of yet
• If you are breast-feeding	• Safety not established as of yet
• If you have severe heart failure	• Patients with severe heart failure had worsening of their heart failure while on etanercept
• If you have tuberculosis	• Etanercept suppresses TNF-alpha and can lead to recurrence of tuberculosis
• If you have any history of recurrent, recent, severe, or current infections	• TNF-alpha suppresses the immune system, which is important in fighting infections
• If you have multiple sclerosis	• Could worsen multiple sclerosis
• If you have a history of liver disease (hepatitis B)	• Could worsen hepatitis

What Side Effects Can Etanercept Cause?

In clinical studies done in psoriasis and psoriatic arthritis, etanercept was generally well tolerated. The most common side effects included:

- reaction at the injection site (redness or swelling); approximately one-third of patients can have an injection site reaction where the skin at the site of injection becomes red and itchy; it will generally go away on its own, but if it progresses, you should contact your doctor
- cold (upper respiratory tract infection)
- headaches
- flu-like symptoms

In the clinical trials, the rates of infection in psoriasis patients were essentially similar between those on etanercept and those receiving a placebo. Serious infections were seen in approximately 1 percent of patients. Reactions at the site of injection were significantly more common in the etanercept group. The reactions were generally mild, and resolved on their own.

Higher rates of lymphoma were reported in patients receiving etanercept. Many of these patients were on other immunosuppressant medication at that time or had been in the past. In addition, they also had other medical conditions, e.g., rheumatoid arthritis. Because these factors could have predisposed them to developing a lymphoma, it is unclear how and if etanercept will increase a patient's risk of lymphoma. Cancers, heart failure, and neurological events were rarely reported in patients taking etanercept. It is not clear how and if etanercept has caused these rare side effects.

How Do You Store Etanercept?

Etanercept is provided in a vial in a dose tray in powder form. After mixing the powder with solution, refrigerate it right away (36°–46°F/2°–8°C). Once a vial of etanercept has been opened, it must be used within the next fourteen days.

It is important to check the expiration date stamped on the carton, dose tray label, and vial label. If any of these labels is past the expiration date, do not use.

Adalimumab (A-da-LIM-u-mab) (Humira®)

This biologic therapy is currently approved in Canada and the U.S. for the treatment of adults with rheumatoid arthritis, psoriatic arthritis, and psoriasis. Adalimumab binds and blocks tumor necrosis factor-alpha (TNF-alpha), a chemical that is made by cells in the immune system and sends faulty signals to the skin and joints. Patients with psoriasis and psoriatic arthritis produce too much TNF-alpha, which results in the inflammation causing red, scaly, skin lesions and swollen, tender joints. Adalimumab helps reduce the inflammation by blocking and reducing the amount of TNF-alpha, and interrupting the inflammatory cycle that is seen in psoriasis and psoriatic arthritis. Adalimumab works quite quickly and many patients will notice an improvement within the first month; however, for others it may take up to three or four months to see the best improvement.

How Is Adalimumab Given?

Adalimumab is a self-administered injection under the surface of the skin. Adalimumab is given as an 80 milligram injection on day one, followed by 40 milligrams every other week, beginning on day eight in patients with psoriasis. The recommended dose for patients with psoriatic arthritis is 40 milligrams every other week.

Your doctor or nurse will give you detailed instructions for preparing and giving an injection. There is also an information package provided with your medication that will have step-by-step instructions. If you have any questions, you can ask your doctor or nurse.

What Results Can You Expect from Adalimumab?
Clinical studies have established that adalimumab showed a rapid and excellent improvement in psoriasis and psoriatic arthritis. Adalimumab was proven to be highly effective in psoriasis studies to date, with 71 percent of patients having an excellent response (75 percent improvement). As seen with other biologic agents, continued treatment can provide additional improvement. Adalimumab has also been used in combination with other types of treatment, such as methotrexate, NSAIDs, or SAARDs in the treatment of psoriatic arthritis.

What should you tell your doctor before starting adalimumab? You should tell your doctor if you:
• are pregnant or plan on becoming pregnant
• are breast-feeding
• have problems with your immune system (i.e., HIV/AIDS)
• have a history of heart failure
• have a history of cancer
• have tuberculosis, have had it, or have recently been exposed to it; you will need to have a tuberculosis skin test done prior to starting adalimumab therapy
• have had recent severe infection, or are prone to infections or recurring infections
• are taking any other medications or herbal supplements
• have an allergy to adalimumab or any of its components
• have problems or diseases with the nervous system, such as multiple sclerosis; if you experience any numbness, tingling, or visual changes before, during or after adalimumab treatment, you should tell your doctor; a small number of patients who have received adalimumab have experienced

a worsening of their multiple sclerosis and other rare diseases of the nervous system (Guillain-Barré, optic neuritis)

What should you tell your doctor while receiving adalimumab? If you develop any of the following while taking adalimumab, you should contact your doctor immediately:

Infections: If you develop an infection or symptoms of an infection, you might need to stop taking adalimumab, so contact your doctor. If your doctor gives you a treatment for infection, it should be taken right away and as prescribed. Treatment with adalimumab should be stopped if you develop a serious infection. Symptoms may include fever, fatigue, and/or a cough. Other symptoms could include a raised, hot, red area of the skin that is spreading. If you feel unwell, but do not have a fever, it is important to tell your doctor. As adalimumab can suppress your immune system, your body may not respond to an infection with a fever as it normally would. If your doctor gives you treatment for an infection, it should be taken right away and as prescribed. The treatment with adalimumab should be stopped if you develop a serious infection.

Symptoms of heart failure: Tell your doctor immediately if you develop new or worsening symptoms of heart failure, such as shortness of breath, swelling of your feet, ankles, or calves.

If you develop cancer: Tell your doctor right away. Adalimumab can suppress the immune system, which is important in fighting cancer.

Vaccination: You should not receive live vaccines while taking adalimumab. Tell your doctor if you need a vaccine.

Who Should Not Take Adalimumab?

Who Should Not Take Adalimumab?	Why
• If you are pregnant or plan on becoming pregnant	• Safety not established as of yet
• If you are breast-feeding	• Safety not established as of yet
• In severe heart failure	• Patients in severe heart failure can experience worsening of their heart failure while on other TNF antagonists
• If you have tuberculosis	• Suppresses TNF-alpha and can lead to recurrence of tuberculosis
• If you have any history of recent, severe, or current infections	• Adalimumab suppresses the immune system, which is important in fighting infections
• If you have multiple sclerosis	• Could worsen multiple sclerosis
• If you have a history of liver disease (i.e., hepatitis B)	• Could worsen hepatitis

What Side Effects Can Adalimumab Cause?

In clinical studies done in psoriasis and psoriatic arthritis, adalimumab was generally well tolerated. The most common side effects included:

- reaction at the injection site (redness or swelling); Approximately one-third of patients can have an injection site reaction where the skin at the site of the injection becomes red and itchy, which will generally go away on its own, but if it progresses, you should contact your doctor
- cold (upper respiratory tract infection)
- headaches
- flu-like symptoms

In the clinical trials, rates of infections in psoriasis patients were essentially similar between those on adalimumab and those receiving a placebo. Serious infections were seen in approximately 1 percent of patients. Reactions at the site of injection were significantly more common in the adalimumab group. The reactions were generally mild, and resolved on their own.

Higher rates of lymphoma were reported in patients receiving adalimumab. Many of these patients were on other immunosuppressive medications at the time or had been on them in the past. In addition, they had other medical conditions, e.g., rheumatoid arthritis. Because these factors could have predisposed them to developing a lymphoma, it is unclear how and if adalimumab will increase the patient's risk of lymphoma. Cancers, heart failure, and neurological events were rarely reported in patients taking adalimumab. It is not clear how and if adalimumab have caused these rare side effects.

How Do You Store Adalimumab?

Adalimumab is provided in prefilled syringes and prefilled pens. Cartons of adalimumab should be refrigerated at 36°–46°F (2°–8°C) and protected from light until the time of administration. It is important not to use adalimumab beyond the expiration date.

Ustekinumab (Us-te-KIN-u-mab) (Stelara®)

Ustekinumab was recently approved in Canada and the U.S. for the treatment of psoriasis, but is not approved for the treatment of psoriatic arthritis. Several large studies have been conducted and research is ongoing regarding its use in psoriatic arthritis.

Ustekinumab is the first of a new class of medications that targets chemical messengers known as interleukin-12 (IL-12) and interleukin-23 (IL-23). These are naturally occurring proteins that are important in regulating the immune system and believed to be associated with certain immune-related inflammatory diseases, such as psoriasis. This new medication regulates IL-12 and IL-23, reducing the inflammation in the skin cells and helping to control the signs and symptoms of psoriasis. Of interest, it is becoming increasingly clear that IL-23 and a new type of recently described T-cell (T-helper 17) are of central importance in the development of psoriasis (see Chapter 2). Interleukin-23 stimulates the growth and the survival of T-helper 17 cells, which may be of central importance in stimulating the skin cell to proliferate, resulting in the changes of psoriasis.

Research trials that have involved targeting interleukin-12 and interleukin-23 have shown some of the highest response rates in the treatment of psoriasis, supporting the central role of these molecules in the cause of psoriasis.

How Is Ustekinumab Given?

Ustekinumab is given by an injection just under the surface of the skin. It is self-administered as a 45 milligram dose administered at week zero, and then week four. It is then given every twelve weeks thereafter. In patients who have a body weight greater than 220 pounds (100 kilograms), 90 milligrams may be used as an alternate dose. For certain patients not responding to this dose, ustekinumab may be given every eight weeks.

Your doctor or nurse will give you detailed instructions for preparing and giving an injection. There is also an information package provided with your medication that will give you step-by-step instructions. If you have any questions, ask your doctor or nurse.

What Can You Expect from Ustekinumab?

Clinical studies have established that ustekinumab has shown an excellent improvement in psoriasis. Research in the use of ustekinumab in psoriatic arthritis is encouraging, but the medication is not yet approved for the treatment of psoriatic arthritis. Ustekinumab is found to be among the most effective treatments in the management of psoriasis with 67–76 percent of patients who received two doses at 45 or 90 milligrams, respectively, at week zero and week four achieving an excellent improvement (75 percent improvement) compared with approximately 3–4 percent of patients receiving a placebo when assessed at 12 weeks after the first injection. Long-term results from these studies have indicated a sustained benefit in the majority of patients.

An additional study compared ustekinumab with etanercept in approximately 900 patients with psoriasis. Two groups of patients received either the 45 or 90 milligram dose of ustekinumab (at weeks zero and four) or the 50 milligram dose of etanercept (received twice weekly during twelve weeks). Study results showed that 68 percent and 74 percent of patients receiving ustekinumab at 45 or 90 milligrams, respectively, achieved an excellent response (75 percent improvement in the Psoriasis Area Severity Index) compared with 57 percent of those patients receiving 50 milligrams of etanercept. The safety profile was similar between these two drugs when examined in the short term, up to 12 weeks. Long-term safety differences between these two drugs, if any, are not known.

As seen with the other biologic agents, continuing to give additional therapy over time can provide additional benefit.

What Should You Tell Your Doctor before Starting Ustekinumab?

You should tell your doctor if you:

- are pregnant or plan on becoming pregnant
- are breast-feeding
- have problems with your immune system (i.e., HIV/AIDS)
- have a history of cancer
- have tuberculosis, have had it, or have recently been exposed to it; you will need to have a tuberculosis skin test done prior to starting ustekinumab therapy
- have had recent severe infection, or are prone to infections or recurring infections
- are taking any other medications or herbal supplements
- have an allergy to ustekinumab or any of its components

In clinical studies done in psoriasis, ustekinumab is generally well tolerated. The most common side effect included upper respiratory tract infections, such as a sinus infection and sore throat, which will usually clear up. If not, consult your doctor.

An uncommon side effect includes cellulitis, a type of infection under the skin. If you develop red, warm discoloration of the skin that is spreading, you should contact your doctor.

How Do You Store Ustekinumab?

Ustekinumab is provided in a vial that should be stored in the refrigerator at 36°–46°F (2°–8°C). The medication is a colorless to light-yellow fluid that may contain a few white particles. If your dose is 45 milligrams, you will receive one 45 milligram vial. If your dose is 90 milligrams, you will receive two 45 milligram vials and will need to give yourself two injections, one right after the other.

Make sure you check the expiration date stamped on the carton. If it is past the expiration date, you cannot use it. In addition, check the vial to make sure that it is not damaged, and the liquid is not cloudy or frozen.

Who Should Not Take Utekinumab?

Who Should Not Take Utekinumab?	Why
• If you are pregnant or plan on becoming pregnant	• Safety not established as of yet
• If you are breast-feeding	• Safety not established as of yet
• If you have tuberculosis	• Safety not established as of yet
• If you have any history of recent, severe or current infections	• Ustekinumab suppresses the immune system, which is important in fighting infections

How Do I Decide Which Biologic Is Right for Me?

The development of a number of new specific, rational therapies has been an important advance in the treatment of psoriasis and has led to an important shift in the way that dermatologists manage this chronic disease. Nonetheless, the number of choices that patients are faced with makes the decision as to which biologic they would choose confusing. Before making a decision, discuss your preferences and thoughts regarding the type of therapy you want with your physician as this will help determine the right choice for you.

There are several questions to consider that may help you decide among the biologics.

• What type of psoriasis do I have?

The biologics have been mostly studied in plaque psoriasis. There have been some preliminary case reports showing the effectiveness of infliximab and adalimumab in some of the other subsets of psoriasis, such as pustular psoriasis.

• Do I have psoriatic arthritis?

The only approved therapies at this time for psoriatic arthritis are etanercept, adalimumab, and infliximab. There have been some preliminary smaller encouraging studies using alefacept and ustekinumab in psoriatic arthritis; however, these drugs are not approved for psoriatic arthritis in Canada.

• How is it given?

Most biologics are self-administered (alefacept, etanercept, adalimumab, and ustekinumab). For patients who wish to self-administer (self-inject) therapies, this would be an important consideration.

For some patients, however, they may prefer to have someone else administer the therapy, such as with infliximab. In this situation, patients go to infusion centers, where they receive therapy over approximately 2 hours. One advantage of these centers is that there are nurses present for counseling, and follow-up of patients is done on a regular basis.

It is expected, however, that if you self-inject (with etanercept, adalimumab, alefacept, or ustekinumab) that you would also follow up regularly in your physician's office. If you have trouble taking medication on a regular basis, or as directed by your physician, this may be a good option for you.

- How often do I receive the medication?
  The frequency of injection varies from once to twice weekly (etanercept) to every two to three months (infliximab and ustekinumab) (see the table for all details).

- What response can I expect?
  It is important to remember that most biologic therapies have not been compared against each other, so it is not possible to directly compare their effectiveness. Still, the response rates from the different studies have been reported and are outlined in the table.

- Is there a reason why I should not receive this drug?
  For each of the drugs, there will be certain patients who should not receive the therapy (contraindication) for specific reasons. These have been outlined in the prior chapter, but some of the key reasons are listed in the table.

The table summarizes some of the main differences between the various biologic agents, and considerations that may help in choosing which biologic is right for you.

---

* Initial infusion given at week zero and day 8

+ Initial infusion given at day zero, week two, and week six

† Initial injections given at day zero and week 4.

• Response rates are short-term results, at weeks 10–16 after beginning therapy, as reported in the major clinical trials. Additional benefit, or loss of benefit, may be experienced over the longer term. Please discuss with your physician.

Biologic Therapies: Which Biologic Is Right for Me?

Therapy	How Does It Work?	How Is It Given?	What Response Can I Expect?	Who Should Not Take It?	Special Considerations
Alefacept (Amevive®)	Anti-T-cell	Injected by a nurse or self-injected into the muscle or just below the skin once a week for twelve weeks	A good response is seen in 42% of patients An excellent response is seen in 21% of patients	People who: • have low T-cell counts • are pregnant or breast-feeding • have serious infections • have HIV/AIDS	• Slower onset of response • May be prolonged periods when patient is disease-free, and no treatment is required
Etanercept (Enbrel®)	Anti-TNF	Self-injected (subcutaneous) once or twice weekly	A good response is seen in 64% receiving 25 mg twice weekly and in 77% receiving 50 mg twice weekly An excellent response is seen in 34–49% of patients	People who: • are pregnant or breast-feeding • have heart failure • have tuberculosis • have recurrent infections • have multiple sclerosis • have liver disease	• Fast onset of response and high response rate • Effective in psoriatic arthritis • Good long-term control • Self-injected once or twice weekly • Established class of drugs with extensive experience in psoriasis and other autoimmune diseases (i.e. rheumatoid arthritis)
Adalimumab (Humira®)	Anti-TNF	Self-injected every two weeks*	A good response is seen in approximately 88% of patients An excellent response is seen in 71% of patients	People who: • are pregnant or breast-feeding • have heart failure • have tuberculosis • have recurrent infections • have multiple sclerosis • have liver disease	• Fast onset of response and high response rate • Likely the highest and fastest response rate among biologics initially • Effective in psoriatic arthritis • Self-injected every two weeks* • Established class of drugs with extensive experience in psoriasis and other autoimmune diseases (i.e. rheumatoid arthritis)
Infliximab (Remicade®)	Anti-TNF	By infusion at infusion center every eight weeks+	A good response is seen in 91% of patients An excellent response is seen in 80% of patients	People who: • are pregnant or breast-feeding • have heart failure • have tuberculosis • have recurrent infections • have multiple sclerosis • have liver disease	• Fast onset of response and high response rate • Intermittent, infrequent dosing every eight weeks+ • Must be given in an infusion center • Effective in psoriatic arthritis • Established class of drugs with extensive experience in psoriasis and other autoimmune diseases (i.e. rheumatoid arthritis)
Ustekinumab (Stelara®)	Anti-IL-12/23	Self-injected every twelve weeks†	A good response is seen in 84% receiving 45 mg and in 89% receiving 90 mg An excellent response is seen in 67–76% of patients	People who: • are pregnant or breast-feeding • have tuberculosis • have recurrent infections	• Intermittent, infrequent dosing every three months • Self-injected every three months.† • New class of drugs targeting a key step in the cause of psoriasis

Side Effects, Reactions and Risks

Common Side Effects
Most common side effects are not serious (see table below).

Injection-Site Reactions
Redness at the drug-injection site has been commonly seen in patients treated with biologics. The majority of the injection-site reactions have been mild (see table below).

Allergic Reactions
Any drug can cause an allergic reaction in some people. See the table below for symptoms.

Side Effects

Common Side Effects	Injection Site Reactions	Allergic Reactions
• nasal congestion • sore throat • fatigue • headache • dizziness	• swelling • pain • bruising • itching • skin irritation • a burning sensation	• fever • chills • hives • rash • shakiness • headache • nausea • flushing • light-headedness • irregular heartbeats • shortness of breath • low blood pressure • difficulty swallowing • difficulty breathing • chest tightness

Infections

Because biologics affect your immune system, you may have an increased risk of developing an infection or having a more severe infection.

The most common infections seen are as follows:
- nasopharyngitis
- upper respiratory tract infections
- bronchitis

The most common type of serious infections seen are as follows:
- pneumonia
- cellulitis
- diverticulitis
- urinary tract infections
- sepsis

Tell your doctor if you have a new infection, if an infection keeps coming back, or if you experience the following:
- fever
- chills
- headache
- coughing
- congestion
- chest tightness
- shortness of breath
- flu-like symptoms
- nausea
- tiredness
- night sweats

- vomiting
- diarrhea
- burning while passing urine
- redness or swelling of skin or joint
- cold sores
- new or worsening of pain in any location
- weight loss

Other Risks

Cancer

Because biologics affect your immune system, you may have an increased risk of developing cancer. In clinical trials, most of the cancers have been non-melanoma skin cancers, which include basal cell or squamous cell carcinomas of the skin, which are usually non-life threatening if caught early. As a precaution, you may wish to limit your sun exposure and undergo regular skin examination skin by a physician when being treating with biologics.

Cardiac and Vascular

People who have psoriasis, and certain other inflammatory diseases, have a higher risk of having heart attacks. These people have heart attacks more often than other people. Seek medical care immediately if you develop the following:
- chest pain or discomfort
- trouble breathing
- irregular heartbeats
- dizziness
- loss of balance
- new numbness or weakness
- visual or speech changes

Pregnancy

The effects of biologics on human sperm and unborn babies is not known. It is very important that women do not become pregnant while being treated with biologics. If you think that you have become pregnant or may have fathered a child while being treated with biologics, tell your doctor immediately.

Tuberculosis

Those who are being treated with biologics may be at a greater risk for serious infections such as tuberculosis. Tell your doctor if you or anyone one in your family has ever had tuberculosis, or if you have ever come in contact with someone with the disease. Tell your doctor if you develop the following:

- a cough that does not go away
- coughing up blood
- shortness of breath
- fever
- night sweats
- weight loss

Vaccinations

Vaccines are made to help protect people from certain illnesses. Some vaccines are made from live bacteria or live viruses. You cannot receive this kind of live vaccine if you are being treated with biologics. Other kinds of vaccines, like tetanus and flu shots, are allowed. Tell your study doctor before getting any vaccine while you are being treated with biologics.

THIRTEEN

Final Thoughts

The past decade has witnessed significant advances in our understanding of the key causes of psoriasis. As a result, novel and highly targeted medications have been developed, and are now becoming available to patients with psoriasis and psoriatic arthritis. Scientific research continues to shed light on the causes of psoriasis and allows for the development of such new therapies to benefit patients.

In the future, it is hoped that developments will evolve in the following major areas.

Increased Understanding of the Causes of Psoriasis

There have been significant advances in our understanding of the key causes of psoriasis. The immune system has been recognized as playing a major role in the formation of psoriasis. This immune dysfunction results in the generation of immune cells (like T-lymphocytes) that release chemical messengers, called cytokines, which stimulate the skin and joints to create the characteristic red, scaling lesions of psoriasis and swollen, tender joints of psoriatic arthritis. Increasing knowledge of the pathways and triggers of inflammation, and the immunologic basis for psoriasis, will enable us to develop specifically targeted biologic agents. It is believed that they will be safer and work more effectively. Currently there are a number of these exciting new drugs under development.

Interleukin-12 (IL-12) and Interleukin-23 (IL-23)

IL-12 and IL-23 have been recently identified as the key chemical messengers (or cytokines) that may act as a switch to turn on the immune abnormalities of psoriasis. Additional studies with drugs that target this pathway are ongoing. Recent studies using antibodies against components of these cytokines and other important cytokines such as IL-22, IL-23 and IL-17 are planned or ongoing and have had striking results and hold major promise as a future treatment of psoriasis.

Genetics and Pharmacogenomics

DNA is found within the heart of the cell and provides the blueprint for a person's makeup, including that of health and disease. Understanding the genetics of psoriasis will provide several benefits. First, doctors will be able to accurately predict who might develop more severe forms of disease and psoriatic arthritis. Second, doctors may be able to develop new therapies that target the genetic abnormality of psoriasis. This will provide a number of benefits:

- Different genes might be involved in different people. New drugs could be developed to target these specific genes.
- Future clinical research could be directed only to patients who will be expected to respond to those certain medications, based on their genetic makeup.
- More accurate calculation of drug dosage will be possible.

Currently, doctors prescribe medications on a trial and error basis. If a certain medication does not work, a doctor might increase the dose, add other medications, or switch medications. If doctors could predict which medications would work best for an individual patient, it would help reduce the trial and error period, decrease the time needed to find an effective therapy, and minimize potential side effects.

Pharmacogenomics could provide doctors with this advantage in the future. The field of pharmacogenomics involves studying how an individual's genetic makeup affects the body's response to different drugs.

Patients with psoriasis are familiar with the concept that what may work for one person may not work for another. In fact, the specific treatments that we often choose in psoriasis are highly individualized to each patient. A number of factors can influence a response to medication, such as environment, diet, age, lifestyle, and health. Of central importance to understanding a person's response to medicine is his or her individual genetic makeup. Understanding this information could provide us with information about which medications might be most beneficial and safe.

- Pharmacogenomics is an exciting area of research that may help scientists and doctors understand why certain patients respond well to particular medications, and to predict to which medications patients will respond to best. Doctors may be able to analyze the genetic profile of a patient and determine the best therapy.

- Also, knowing a patient's genetic profile could help determine the best dose rather than the traditional method of giving a fixed dose to each patient or basing it solely on his or her weight.

Understanding which patients might be expected to respond to a medication would help in choosing the most effective treatment. Also, it could be possible to determine which patients might have certain severe side effects, which are always of great concern to doctors and patients alike.

Determining Prognosis

At present, we are unable to accurately determine which children or adults will progress to more severe disease or develop psoriatic arthritis. Ultimately, understanding the genetic makeup of an individual and the key determinants of psoriasis could enable us to predict which patients will progress to more severe disease or psoriatic arthritis. This might permit the early introduction of certain medications or changes in lifestyle/environmental to minimize the impact of this disease.

In short, pharmacogenomics may enable us to predict the best medication for specific patients for improved benefit in their disease and safety in their overall health.

Final Thoughts

One of the most exciting areas in the field of psoriasis is the increasing understanding of the causes of the disease and the development of new medicines that can target these abnormalities in the immune system. The complex yet fascinating interplay between genetics, environmental triggers, and the immune system that result in psoriasis and psoriatic arthritis continue to be determined. Such advances have provided scientists with the ability to develop novel treatments, which are translating into improved choices for patients and their families. While these advances continue, it is hoped that the "heartbreak of psoriasis" will be reduced or eliminated, and that psoriasis will become a disease that is diagnosed and controlled easily, using safer and effective therapies.

Table of Drug Names

Generic Name	Common Brand Name
Photosensitizing Medications	
Amiodarone	Cordarone®
Amitriptyline	Elavil®
Atenolol	Tenoretic®
Captopril	Capoten®
Chlorpromazine	Thorazine®
Ciproflaxacin	Cipro®
Coal tar	Estar®, Balnetar®
NSAIDs	e.g., Desipramine®, Diclofenac®, Ibuprofen®, aprosyn®
Diltiazem	Cardizern®
Doxycycline	Vibramycin®
Ecalapril	Vasotec®
Thiazide diuretic	
Etretinate	Tegison®
Fluorouracil	Adrucil®
Furosemide	Lasix®
Glyburide	Diabeta®
Griseofulvin	Fulvicin U/F®
Hydralazine	Apresoline-Esidrix®
Hydrochlorothiazide	Hydrodiuril®
Labetalol	Normodyne®
Lisinopril + Hydrochlorothiazide	
Lovastatin	Mevacor®
Minocycline	Minocin®
Nadolol + Bendroflumethiazide	Corzide®
Nifedipine	Adalat®
Norfloxacin	Noroxin®
Phenytoin	Dilantin®
Spironolactone + Hydrochlorothiazide	
Sulfasalazine	Azulfidine®
Tetracycline	Sumycin®
Thioriclazine	
Tretinoin	Retin-A®
Trimethoprim	Bactrim®, Septra®
NSAIDs	
Celecoxib: Cox-2	Celebrex®
Diclofenac	Arthrotec®
Ibuprofen	Advil®, Motrin®
Indomethacin	Indocid®
Ketoprofen	Orudis SR®, Rhodis®, Rhovail®
Naproxen	Naprosyn®
Salicylate	Aspirin®
Tolmetin	Tolectin®

Glossary

Abscess: A localized collection of pus.

Acitretin: A vitamin A-like drug, or retinoid, taken by mouth for the treatment of psoriasis.

Acute: Severe and quick onset of a disease or disorder.

AIDS: Acquired immune deficiency syndrome, a disease caused by the human immunodeficiency virus, which causes the body to have decreased immune capacity (i.e., the ability to fight infections).

Anthralin: A topical medication used to treat psoriasis; may be used alone or in combination with ultraviolet light (Ingram regimen).

Antibody: A protein produced by the immune system cells that binds to antigens so other elements of the immune system can attack and destroy or remove the antigen.

Antigen: A large molecule or small organism whose entry into the body provokes an immune-system response; a foreign substance, usually a protein, which causes the formation of an antibody.

Apoptosis: Death of cells by a controlled mechanism.

Arachidonic acid: A fatty acid found in high levels in the skin of patients with psoriasis that could contribute to inflammation and cell growth.

Atrophy: Thinning of the skin.

Autoimmune disease: A condition in which the body produces antibodies against itself (autoantibodies); that is, they attack the body's own cells and disrupt normal bodily functions.

Biologic agents: Biologics are made from living cells and are designed to target specific steps in the disease process. Biologics are proteins that are injected subcutaneously, intramuscularly, or intravenously.

Biopsy: The removal of a small piece of body tissue for examination under a microscope (e.g., a skin biopsy).

Biotechnology: A set of techniques, such as those used to make DNA in laboratories, developed through basic research that are now used by companies to make new drugs.

Calcipotriol: A synthetic form of vitamin D3 used in the treatment of psoriasis.

Cell: The basic structural and functional unit of living organisms; a cell contains the genetic information; a cell nucleus contains twenty-three pairs of chromosomes (one half of each pair is inherited from each parent).

Chromosome: Each chromosome contains thousands of individual genes, which give people their distinct characteristics; genetic information is encoded in long strands of a chemical called deoxyribonucleic acid (DNA), which is shaped in two connected strands that look like a twisted ladder (called a double helix).

Chronic: Long lasting.

Clinical trial phases:
- Phase I: The earliest type of trials, which are usually done on normal, healthy volunteers
- Phase II: Early trials in which specific doses are tested to see which is the most effective, and to test for safety

- Phase III: Large trials that are conducted before the drug becomes approved; safety and effectiveness of the drug are tested in this phase

Corticosteroid: A topical medication helpful in treating psoriasis. Topical steroids come in different strengths (i.e., mild, moderate, potent, very potent) and formulations (cream, ointment, lotion). If corticosteroids are given orally, psoriasis may improve, but it will often worsen or flare up when the medication is ceased. Oral steroids are seldom used to treat psoriasis.

Cyclosporine: An immunosuppressive drug best known for preventing rejection of transplanted organs; also a psoriasis systemic treatment.

Cytokine: Proteins used by the immune system to communicate messages among cells; in psoriasis, cytokines send faulty signals that promote inflammation and the overly rapid development of skin cells.

Dermatologist: A doctor who has undergone extensive training in the diagnosis and treatment of diseases of the skin, hair, and nails after completing medical school.

Dermis: The layer of skin just below the epidermis.

Distal interphalangeal joints (DIP): The joints of the ends of fingers closest to the nails.

DNA: Abbreviation of deoxyribonucleic acid. DNA carries genetic information in each cell.

Epidermis: The outermost, superficial layers of the skin. The epidermis is made up of an outer dead layer (stratum corneum) and a deeper, living cellular zone (spinous layer, basal layer). The epidermis rests on (epi = on top of) the dermis.

Etretinate: An older form of a vitamin A (retinoid) drug used to treat psoriasis.

Flexural psoriasis: Also known as inverse psoriasis, affecting the folds of skin in the armpits, groin, and/or genitalia.

Genes: Genes are arranged like beads on a string; they are short sections of DNA that hold the recipe for a specific protein or molecule; the recipe is spelled out by the arrangement of four chemicals that connect the strands of DNA in pairs (called base pairs).

Gene therapy: The injection of healthy genes into the bloodstream for the purpose of treating a hereditary disease.

Goeckerman regimen: A regime combining crude coal tar and ultraviolet light for the treatment of psoriasis.

Home phototherapy: The use of an ultraviolet light source at home to treat skin diseases such as psoriasis.

Immune deficiency: A deficiency in the immune system that may be acquired (AIDS) or inherited (i.e., SCID).

Inflammation: The immune system's protective reaction or response to injury or infection, characterized by pain, swelling, redness, heat, and sometimes loss of function.

Interferons: Originally described as proteins formed when cells are exposed to a virus. Now they are recognized for their important role in the development of psoriasis.

Interleukin: A type of cellular messenger (or cytokines) that stimulates the growth and maturation of cells of the immune system.

Keratinocyte: A type of skin cell. The accelerated growth of these cells leads to the development of the thick, scaly skin of psoriasis.

Keratolytic: A topical medication that promotes the shedding of the epidermis (i.e., salicylic acid).

Koebner phenomenon: Describes the formation of psoriasis at the site of an injury or trauma.

Lesion: A term that denotes an abnormality in the skin, as when an area of skin is affected by psoriasis.

Macrophage: Also called antigen-presenting cells (APCs) because they present antigens to T-cells, macrophages destroy foreign antigens and initiate T-cell formation.

Maintenance therapy: Therapy that is continued after clearance or near clearance of the disease in order to maintain clearance or near clearance.

Methotrexate: A chemotherapy-like drug used in the treatment of psoriasis; given once weekly by mouth or intramuscular injection.

Monotherapy: Using only one drug to treat psoriasis.

Narrow-band UVB: Ultraviolet light in a narrow band of 311–312 nanometers, which may be more effective in treating psoriasis, and may be less likely to cause skin cancer.

Necrosis: Death or decay of part or all of an organ or tissue due to disease, injury, or deficiency of nutrients.

Ostraceous: Resembling an oyster shell in appearance.

Papule: A raised lesion less than 3/8 inch (1 centimeter) in diameter.

PASI: Psoriasis Area and Severity Index, a measure used in psoriasis clinical trials that examines the body area affected and severity of the disease. Studies usually measure this at the beginning and end of treatment to determine the effect of the medication (PASI-50; PASI-75).

PASI-50: A 50 percent reduction in the PASI; considered to be a significant improvement by patients and physicians.

PASI-75: A 75 percent reduction in the PASI; this is a major improvement in psoriasis with near clearance of lesions; a stringent measure often required by the Federal Drug Administration in the U.S. for the approval of new psoriasis medication.

Photochemotherapy: Refers to the addition of drugs to enhance the effects of ultraviolet light (such as PUVA).

Phototherapy: The use of ultraviolet light (UVA or UVB) to treat disease.

Plaque: A scaly, raised area formed on the skin, which is greater than 3/8 inch (1 centimeter) in diameter.

Pruritic: Itching.

Psoralen: A drug taken orally or applied topically that can increase the effectiveness of ultraviolet-A therapy. It is used in combination with ultraviolet-A to treat psoriasis (PUVA = psoralen plus UVA).

Pus: Yellowish-white fluid formed in infected or noninfected tissue, consisting of white blood cells, cellular debris, and necrotic tissue.

Pustule: A small, raised area of the skin containing pus.

PUVA: Psoralen plus ultraviolet-A light therapy; can be applied topically or systemically.

Red blood cells: Blood cells responsible for carrying oxygen around the body.

Remission: The period during which the symptoms and signs of a disease decrease or subside.

Rheumatologist: A specialist in the treatment of arthritis and related diseases.

Skin biopsy: Taking a small sample of skin with a special instrument (punch biopsy) or a surgical blade for examination under a microscope.

Stratum: Layer; e.g., stratum basale (base layer of skin cells in the epidermis).

Stressors: A stimulus that causes stress.

Striae: Stretch marks.

Symptom: Something abnormal perceived by the patient, such as fatigue, pain, or itch.

Systemic: Affecting the entire body internally.

Systemic lupus erythematosus: Autoimmune disease that causes skin inflammation and can affect multiple organs.

Tachyphylaxis: The development of tolerance to the effects of a drug.

Tars: Natural, sticky substances used to treat psoriasis.

Tazarotene: Vitamin A-like topical medication for the treatment of psoriasis.

T-cells: Immune cells that either initiate the immune response (helper T-cells) or destroy foreign cells (killer T-cells).

T-cell receptors: Molecules on the surface of T-cells that are the sites for antigen-presenting cells to present antigens to the T-cell. In doing so, they teach T-cells to recognize the antigen and can then induce an immune response.

Topical: A medication applied directly to the skin, such as a cream, ointment, or lotion.

UVL: Ultraviolet light.

Vitamin D3: A vitamin, also known as calcipotriol, that is applied topically to treat psoriasis.

White blood cell: Immune cells in the blood that play a role in fighting infection as a part of the immune system.

Further Resources

Organizations

Canada

Amevive Care Program (AWARE)
1-877-263-8483

Arthritis Society
393 University Avenue
Suite 1700
Toronto, ON
M5G 1E6
1-800-321-1433
www.arthritis.ca

Canadian Dermatology Association
1385 Bank Street
Suite 425
Ottawa, ON
K1H 8N4
1-800-267-3376
www.dermatology.ca

Canadian Skin Patient Alliance
2446 Bank Street
Suite 383
Ottawa, ON
KIV 1A8
1-613-422-4265
www.skinpatientalliance.ca

Enbrel Support Program (ENLIVEN)
1-877-936-2735
www.enbrel.ca

Humira Support Program (Progress)
1-866-HUMIRA
1-866-848-6472
www.humira-progress.ca

Remicade Support Program (Bioadvance)
1-877-704-4474

Stelara Support Program (Spectrum)
1-877-705-0555

United States

American Academy of Dermatology
P.O. Box 4014
Schaumburg, IL 60168-4014
1-888-462-DERM
www.aad.org

National Psoriasis Foundation
6600 S.W. 92nd Avenue
Suite 300
Portland, OR 97223-7195
1-800-723-9166
www.psoriasis.org

Books

Cram, D.L. *Coping with Psoriasis: A Patient's Guide to Treatment*. Omaha, NE: Addicus Books, 2000.

Lowe, Nicholas J. *Psoriasis: A Patient's Guide*. London: Infora Health Care, 2003.

Index